New Ways to Cure Acne

"Discover the latest way you can be free of acne and end up with excellent health"

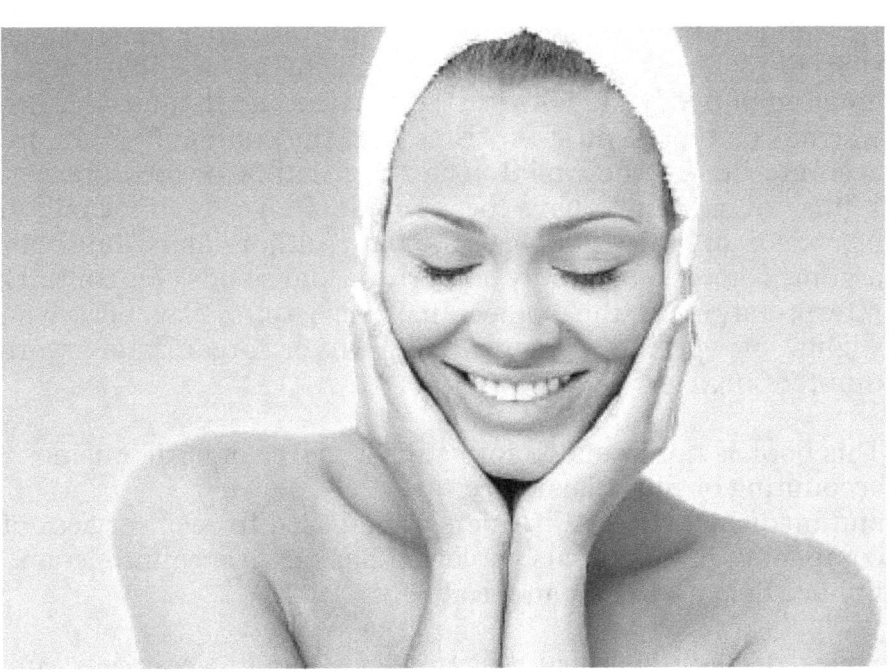

By Christopher Teller, Natural Nutritionist

Table of Content

Chapter 1: What This Book is About

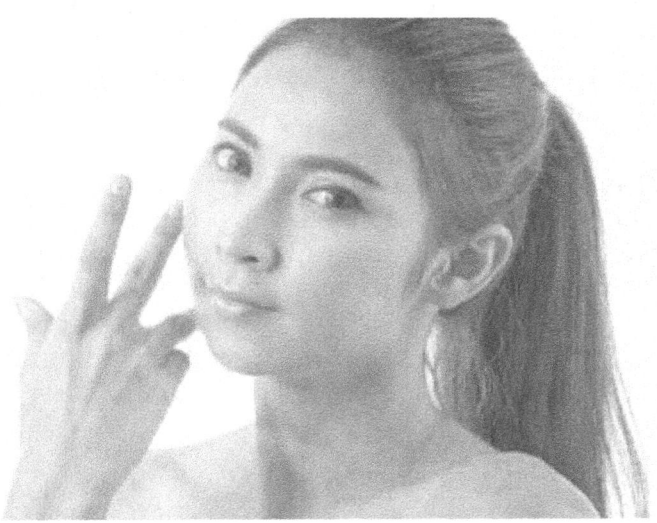

Introduction

In this acne book, you will discover many ways that you can minimize or eliminate your acne problems. Getting rid of acne is not always easy. For some of you, you need only do a few of the recommended techniques listed here. Yet for others you will need to use many until you find what works for you.

The following information is a result of many years of testing and research. It is a fantastic health program that will help you reduce or eliminate acne. Some parts of this program are take a while before you see results. And, you will be tempted to quit and stop before you get acne relief. However, if you want an acne-free face, then you need to be consistent and keep at it until you achieve what you want.

Each chapter has powerful information on how your body

works in creating your acne, and what you need to do to stop and clear that acne. You may experience information overload, But in the end, you will see what you need to do, to have the beauty that was intended for you to have.

In one of the chapters, you will be given a day by day action plan, which you can use for many weeks. There are many ways to do this step by step program. You choose what is best for your situation.

There are many products you can buy, to help you overcome your acne. But, you don't have to buy all of them. You will choose the ones that you want to buy. You will want to choose those that pertain to your acne and health.

I am here to support you and available to provide answers when things are not as clear, as you should like.

Acne Is a Symptom

Acne is a positive symptom that tells you your health is in danger. When you fight your acne, you are fighting to recover your health. So, you have to be strong and aggressive with what you do, to get rid of it.

You can't have a weak approach, when trying to get rid of acne. You have to overdo and be persistent in everything you try. You have to fight hard with the applications in this book, because it not just about acne, but about regaining health inside and out.

Are You Ready to Start?

This is a program that requires motivation and persistent. As with anything that is important and that you want to achieve, it takes hard work.

I can't promise you a two or four-week cure for your acne, but I'll be happy to show you what it takes to eliminate your acne. However, you need to be dedicated to following some strong basic nutritional and health principles. These nutrition principles are the foundation for good clear skin and, better yet, for good active health.

Hi, my name is Christopher Teller nutritional consultant that will be helping you get rid of your acne. I was train in California on how to help people with a variety of diseases. I'm ready to help you.

In This Book

In this book, you find out what acne is all about, and how you can deal with it in a natural and healing way. This book is not about creating a miracle, where you will eliminate your acne in three days or less.

It is about applying known body cleansing techniques and nutritional and herbal remedies that give you better health and facial skin. The way you look and the way you think is a reflection of your body's health. If you have good health or bad health, it will be reflected on your face, physical appearance and your thoughts.

Are You Motivated?

If you are serious and motivate about getting rid of acne, then this book will give you all the details you need. The things you need to do for acne are not easy, but they work, if you are persistent. I cannot guarantee that next week you will be free of acne. The amount of work you put into clearing your acne will determine how quickly you get rid of acne.

Did You Inherit Acne?

If your acne is heredity, it is not true that you cannot do anything about it. If you know that other members of your family have had acne and previous generations also, then you are susceptible to acne. Knowing this, you can now arm yourself with some powerful nutritional and hygiene habits that will prevent acne from taking hold and remaining for what can seem like forever.

How to Start

Go through the chapters, so that you can get familiar with the information and techniques presented. As you continue to review this information, at some point all of this information will become clear to you, as to what it takes to get rid of your acne.

Chapter 2: Hair Follicles Working

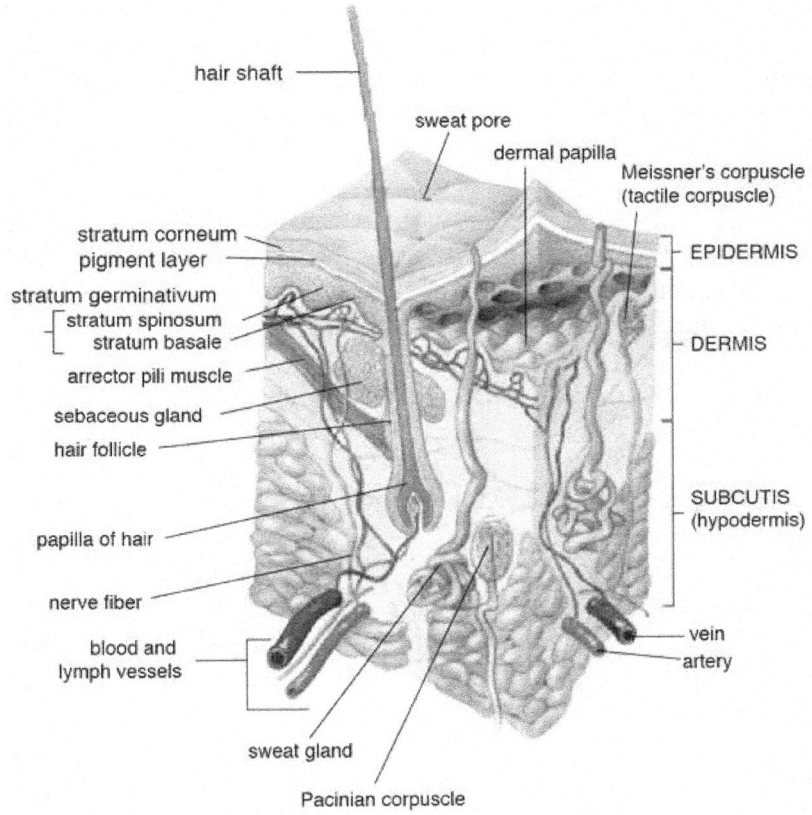

hair shaft

sweat pore

dermal papilla

Meissner's corpuscle
(tactile corpuscle)

stratum corneum

pigment layer

stratum germinativum
stratum spinosum
stratum basale

arrector pili muscle

sebaceous gland

hair follicle

papilla of hair

nerve fiber

blood and
lymph vessels

EPIDERMIS

DERMIS

SUBCUTIS
(hypodermis)

vein

artery

sweat gland

Pacinian corpuscle

Skin an Elimination Channel

Your skin is an elimination channel. It gets rid of extra toxins that come to it, through your blood. It also gets rid of toxins in the tissue that surround your hair follicles that were stored there by your liver.

When all of your elimination organs are working well, your skin has a minimum of toxins to release onto your skin surface. When this happens, your skin will not have plugged pores, inflammation, or acne.

Functions of our Skin

Your skin has many functions. It protects you from the invasion of pathogens. It helps to regulate your body's temperature and controls the amount of body fluids loss during sweating. Your skin protects your body from losing nutrients through it surface.

Your skin provides a way for you to synthesis vitamin D, which is then routed to your small intestine for absorption. At the small intestine, vitamin D helps to transport calcium through your intestinal wall and into your blood.

Your skin is filled with pores and follicles some grow hair and others don't.

Pores in your Skin

Every follicle has a corresponding pore on your face. The pore is an opening on your skin and a shaft that leads past your pore opening. Your follicles consist of a hair shaft or papilla of hair and a bulb or papilla at the bottom of the pore. Along the side of the follicle is the sebaceous gland.

Whether this follicle grows hair is based on the intensity of the hormones you have. For men, testosterone is the dominant hormone, which defines hair growth from facial follicles. For women, estrogen suppresses the growth of facial hair.

It's through the bulb or papilla where your hair shaft is connected to blood vessels that provide it with nutrients, hormones, fatty acids, and toxic matter.

In the diagram below, you see the entire hair follicle structure.

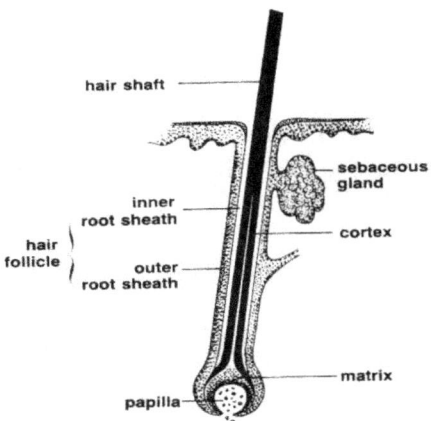

To keep your skin moisturized, your pores have a sebaceous gland, which releases sebum, an oily substance, onto the surface of your skin. Dirt, oil, dead skin cells, and other contaminates collect on your skin, which can plug up your pores.

You need to wash your face, at the end of the day, with Glycerin soap, to keep your skin pores from plugging up. Avoid commercial soaps that have a lot of petrochemicals in their ingredients, to avoid getting them into your blood.

Sebaceous Gland

The sebaceous gland is a tiny gland found in each follicle, which produces odorless sebum. This sebum is a yellowish and waxy substance. It is oily and can keep your skin and hair from drying.

In the sebaceous glands, certain cells produce sebum. When these cells fill up, they burst releasing the sebum, which travels to the skin surface, through the follicle and pore opening.

The sebum consists of triglyceride oils, glycerides, cholesterol, waxes, fatty acids, squalenes (a hydrocarbon), vitamin E, and dead cells. This sebum is odorless, unless it contains bacteria.

Over production of Sebum

A pimple is created, when a pore becomes clogged through harden sebum and dead cells. A pore can also be clogged when excess sebum is created. When a pore becomes clogged, a pimple can form.

Here are some reasons for over the production of sebum.

Menopause – can cause a burst of sebum production for a short time.

Puberty – is a time when hormones are high and cause excess sebum secretions.

Men – tend to produce more sebum than women.

Genetics – is also a factor in over production of sebum. If parents or grandparents had oily faces and scalps, their children could have inherited this trait.

Nutrition – can also contribute to excess sebum. Eating excess fatty food, affects liver function and hormonal balance, which can lead to sebum over production.

Supplements for Normal Sebum Production

Nutrition is the center of controlling the production of sebum oil. It is natural nutrition that gives your body the nutrients it needs, to function properly. When your body becomes unhealthy, illness and sickness can occur in all parts of your body. Then, various organs and body systems function below normal levels.

Vitamin A

Vitamin A lowers excess production of sebum. You can take a supplement to provide you with a good amount of this vitamin. In addition, you can eat foods high in vitamin A, such as carrots, spinach, cheese, and cantaloupes.

Vitamin B

Vitamin B helps to produce the normal levels of sebum. Use a good the multi-vitamin B50 or B100. Eat foods such as fish, green leafy vegetables, and eggs. All recommended diets in this book provide you with the vitamin A and B that you need to control your sebum levels. Most likely, you lack the B vitamins, so supplement with them.

When you don't produce enough sebum, your skin becomes dry. When you produce too much sebum, your skin is oily, and you're prone to acne.

Plugged Pores

There are many other reasons for plugged pores. If you don't keep your skin clean, with the right soap, contaminants, dirt and dead cells can accumulate on your skin, plugging the top opening of your pores. When this happens, sebum cannot reach your skin surface, which then leads to acne.

Chapter Summary

Here are the main points from this chapter. They are the key ideas that you will be using in this program.

Your skin is filled with pores that lead to a follicle tube. It is in your follicles where sebum is produced and where the sebaceous gland exists. It is this gland that releases sebum to prevent your skin from drying and protect it from the sun and bacteria.

When you produce too much sebum, your pores will plug up and cause pimples. Your pores or follicles can become plugged, when you enter puberty or Menopause. Your pores also become plugged, when your hormones are out of balance or when you don't keep your face clean.

Using vitamin A and B50 or B100, will help you to control your sebaceous gland, from releasing too much sebum.

Chapter 3: Acne Disease

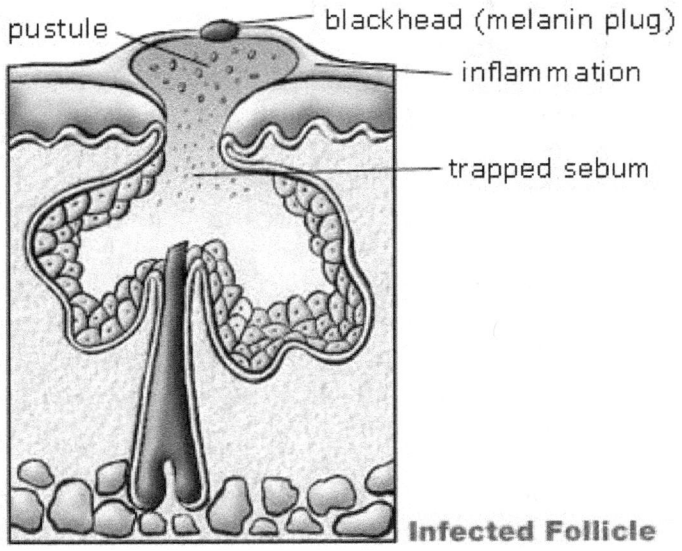

pustule — blackhead (melanin plug)

inflammation

trapped sebum

Infected Follicle

A word of Caution: If you experience sudden face or body eruptions, this can indicate a potentially serious medical condition. If your blemishes look large and like welts, you might want to see your doctor immediately.

Traditional Medical Acne Treatments

There are many traditional treatments that you can use, to give your facial skin some help – medical and natural.

But here are some products you should know about and their effects on your skin.

- Benzoyl peroxide – opens pores to kill bacteria

- Antibiotics – erythromycin, tetracycline, clindamycin – kill bacteria everywhere it goes into your body and skin.

- Retin A – helps to break open plugged pores, prevents new plugged pores, and scarring.

- Topical steroid, cortisone derivatives, drugs help to kill bacteria and control inflammation.

Benzoyl Peroxide   Facial Clean Using Benzoyl Peroxide

There is a lot of controversy concerning the use of benzoyl peroxide to treat acne. In Chapter **25:** Facial Clean Using Benzoyl Peroxide , benzoyl peroxide is used with salicylic acid. This cleansing process is an effective method, for getting rid of acne breakouts. But, if there is a concern on your part with using this facial cleansing method, Chapter **26: Acne Facial Method** is what you should use.

Skin Discoloration

Benzoyl peroxide can cause skin discoloration on moderate to dark skins. Benzoyl creates free radicals in your skin, which slows acne healing. It turns pimples into brown or dark spots as part of the healing process. These dark spots are acne infections that may fade with time, on some people.

When a plugged pimple ruptures, this is how skin scaring takes place. White blood cells rush in to digest collagen around the pore walls. It is these ruptured follicle walls that create inflammation and promote the creation of excess melanin causing skin discoloration.

This is why it is important to be taking zinc, in this program. **Zinc helps** to control the production of melanin.

Benzoyl peroxide can be an effective product to use, to start the cleansing of your face. However, it is not something to use long term, because of its side effects and its skin harshness.

People have reported changes in their overall skin color, when it has been used for years. In this program, you will only use Benzoyl peroxide for a few weeks.

Sunscreen

After using a benzoyl treatment, you can minimize the dark spots on your face by using a broad-spectrum sunscreen, before you go outside. Apply a sunscreen of SPF 30 or higher that is non-comedogenic. This type of sunscreen will not clog your pores. Exposing your skin to the sun without sunscreen causes an excess production of melanin, which makes infected acne areas darker.

Antibiotics

Antibiotics are becoming less effective on acne, because of their overuse. Using only antibiotics to control or eliminate acne has been found not to work for most people. However, there are some people where an antibiotic has helped them to control follicle and facial bacteria.

When antibiotics are combined with anti-inflammatory supplements, Anacin, their acne effectiveness improves. Antibiotics and drugs have serious side effects that you will want to avoid. A treatment for acne with antibiotics must be followed up with probiotics, for at least one month. This is done to replace the good bacteria that were killed by the antibiotics. If this is not done, your bad bacterial will dominate, throughout your body. In addition, your digestion, absorption, and elimination of food will be compromised.

Natural Recommendations

All of my recommendations are natural ways for eliminating acne, except for the first acne facial method, which uses glycolic acid, benzoyl peroxide, and salicylic acid. However, these creams will help to reduce the inflammation and infections on your skin.

Chapter Summary

Here are the main points from this chapter.

Acne is a disease of your sebaceous glands in your follicles. Your glands malfunction, when your pores get plugged with dead cells, dirt, DHT, body toxic matter, and excess sebum oil. When this happens, P-acnes bacteria come into play and multiple, causing plugged pores to enlarge and appear as a pimple on your skin.

Body toxic matter is delivered to your follicles from all parts of your body through your blood stream. Toxic matter also comes into your follicles from the contaminated fat surrounding your follicles.

Facial scars are created, when you have a plugged follicle pore burst. This causes your immune system to remove some of the collagen along the pore wall. This results in a scar and becomes visible, when your plugged pore opens and releases its contaminated contents.

There are a variety of different types of acne that you may develop. But, what is important is that acne is a condition that lets you know that your body is out of balance and in poor health.

Chapter 4: How Your Body Creates Acne

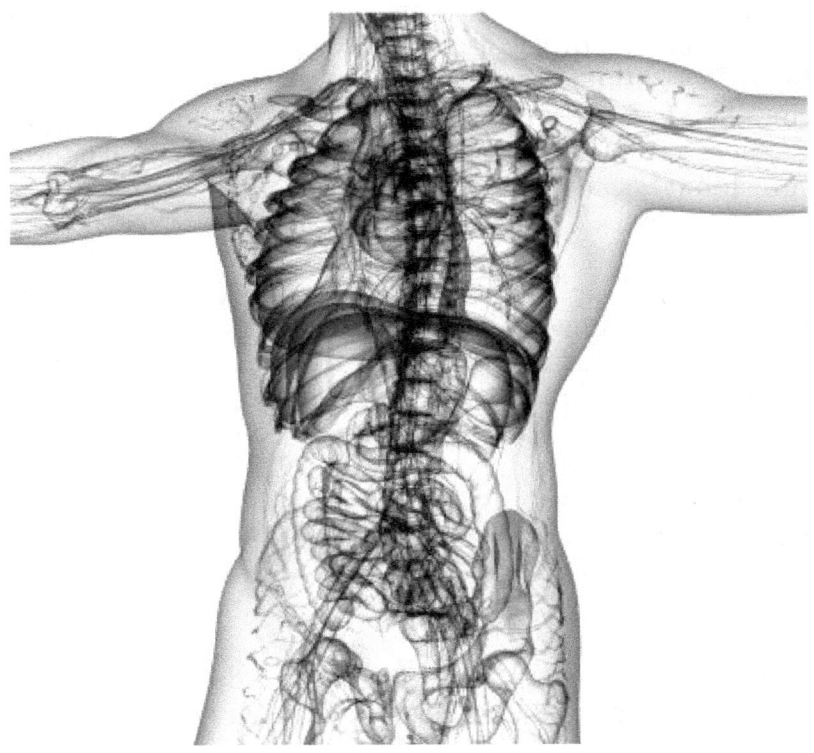

Basic Causes of Acne

To clear your acne permanently, you need to get to the cause.

There can be one or many causes. These causes can depend on your diet, emotional history,
and genetics. There can be many other causes, but when you follow a health program that deals with the whole body, all body imbalances will become balanced.

Yes, you can work on your face with various cream, topological drugs, or washes. This will give you some relief and may even eliminate your facial acne. However, if the cause of your acne is not eliminated, pimples will keep coming back.

The actual cause of acne comes from internal organs or body systems that are overworked and cannot function correctly. This causes your body systems to let excess toxin and hormones get into your blood, instead of being eliminated. The result is that these toxins and hormones can accumulate in your follicles causing them to become plugged and enlarged.

What is Acne?

What is acne? Acne is a skin condition that frequently shows up on your face as an inflamed area called a pimple or a blemish that is filled with bacteria, oil, dead skin cells, and other toxic material. As this inflamed area
progresses, it can continue to grow, until it bursts, or you burst it. Deep scaring can result, if you scratch it, pick at it, or prevent it from healing on its own.

Hormones

Hormones or androgens that are released during puberty and menstrual periods and that exist in adults are one of the major causes of acne. However, because acne is a complex problem, hormones usually are not the sole cause.

Teenager Acne

Acne in teenagers is typically caused by an increase in their sex hormones, androgens. These hormones cause increase sebum production in the follicles. When pores become clogged with dead cells, dirt, and excess sebum, bacteria starts to multiple. This causes white blood cells to rush in to fight the bacteria. The result is a pimple is formed.

Adult Acne

When hormones get completely out of balance, increase sebum occurs in adults. The hormones responsible for adult acne are testosterone, estrogen, dihydrotestosterone, **DHT**, insulin-like growth factor, and dehydroepiandrosterone sulfate, DHEAS.

Testosterone in excess is converted to **DHT** through an enzyme known as 5-alpha reductase. It is **DHT** that activates the sebaceous gland to release more sebum, which leads to acne breakouts.

Women who have polycystic ovary syndrome produce excess testosterone, which is then converted to the acne harmful **DHT**.

When you are stressed, fearful, or angry, your adrenal glands release too much dehydroepiandrosterone sulfate or DHEAS. This hormone converts to testosterone and then to the acne harmful **DHT**. Again excess **DHT** is responsible for activating the sebaceous gland to produce too much sebum, which then leads to acne.

Acne is typical not seen in adults, but when it happens, this acne may be associated with an underlying condition, such as pregnancy, polycystic ovary syndrome, hirsutism or Cushing' syndrome, insulin resistance, poor diet, and emotional conditions.

Polycystic Ovary Syndrome

In difficult cases of acne, the cause may be polycystic ovary syndrome, PCOS. Women with acne, which is hard to eliminate should check with their doctor for this condition.

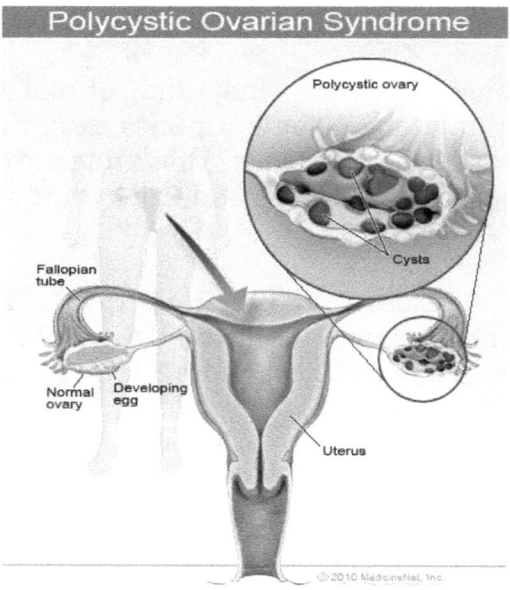

Polycystic ovary syndrome is a condition where some women have enlarged ovaries, with many small cysts along the edge of the ovaries.

When this syndrome is active, women may have prolonged menstrual periods, obesity, acne, or excess hair growth. In cases where no egg is release, women are still able to have a period. Other symptoms are,

- Infertility
- Obesity
- Not able to ovulate
- Absence of menstruation
- Infrequent or light menstruation
- Irregular menstruation
- Excess facial hair
- Excess bleeding

- Elevated levels of male's hormones
- Oily skin or dandruff
- Skin discolorations
- High cholesterol or blood pressure

Causes of Polycystic ovary syndrome (PCOS)

The pituitary gland controls most of the hormonal glands in your body. The hypothalamus controls the pituitary gland. Malfunction of the hypothalamus or pituitary gland is one of the causes of hormonal imbalances leading to acne. These malfunctions can be inherited.

PCOS is also caused by high blood sugar levels, which results in insulin resistance and elevated blood insulin levels. This high insulin may account for the excess amount of male hormones, testosterone, found in PCOS.

Another cause of PCOS may be in a low level of chronic inflammation in your body. Normally, you are not able to feel low levels of inflammation. Low level inflammation is always present in everyone's body, and it's this inflammation that over time creates devastating diseases.

Hirsutism

Hirsutism is a condition that both woman and men can have. When androgens become active in puberty, excess hair can develop in women, where hair normally does not occur, such as in the face, chest, or back.

Hirsutism is caused by an increased level in male hormones or by hair follicles that are over sensitivity to male hormones. The male hormone testosterone stimulates hair growth, increases muscles, deepens the voice, and creates acne in men and women.

Using birth control pills, such as desogestrel, norgestimate or drospirenone, can offset the effects of male androgens and reduce the creation of testosterone, by the ovaries.

If you have hirsutism, it is best to work with your doctor, to eliminate this condition.

Toxins and Acne

Simply, an excess of toxins does not produce acne. There is always toxic matter in your follicle pores. It is this toxic matter with excess sebum that feeds the bacteria in your pores, which results in inflammation and acne.

Acne and Heredity

If your family and ancestors had various weaknesses of skin or of the channel of elimination, which caused acne, then you to might be susceptible to acne.

If you couple susceptibility to acne with excess hormones and toxins, then you set the stage, for forming mild to severe acne.

Does Diet Cause Acne?

Many doctors and researchers are still on the fence on whether diet causes acne. They say,

"The relationship between diet and acne is not very clear. There is no quality evidence that diet creates acne."

However, there is no disease in your body that is not related to your diet. Your body runs on food. If you don't eat the food that your body needs for good health, you will get sick.

Everyone doesn't need to eat the same food to be healthy. Every person can eat differently from another and still be healthy, provided his food is nutritious.

Now there are some diseases that are hereditary or are formed in the womb or during birth and are unrelated to diet. Basically, when you are born with good health, and you develop a disease, it will be related to what you have eaten.

Insulin and Acne

Studies have been made that show when you eat a diet of simple carbohydrates, sugar or high glycemic food, you are more prone to having acne. Drinking milk regularly has also been shown to create or make acne worse.

High glycemic diets tend to make you gain weight and obesity has been associated with acne.

If you have diabetes or are insulin resistance, this condition tends to produce more testosterone, which eventually ends up as DHT.

If you are extra sensitive to testosterone, you can have frequent acne breakouts. This happens because your hormone sebaceous' receptors are over eager to trap testosterone, when it is nearby and immediately convert it to DHT.

Free Radicals

Free radicals formed in the sebaceous glands are involved in the inflammation of your follicles. These free radicals are an added factor that is involved, during the formation of acne. If you have good health, then these radicals are neutralized by antioxidant enzymes such as Superoxide dismutase, SOD, catalase, CAT, glutathione, and others.

If you don't have good health, then you will be lacking these antioxidant enzymes, and your acne will become more inflamed than normal.

The antioxidants supplements that you need are selenium

vitamin A, C, and E, beta carotene, and zinc. All fruits are filled with antioxidants. Antioxidants are found in the different color fruits and vegetables. The more fruits and vegetables you eat the more antioxidants your will get into your body. Antioxidants are what you need, to help you eliminate follicle inflammation, which is associated with acne.

Channels of Elimination

Let's first look at how toxic matter is created and handled by your body. Your body has seven channels of elimination and detoxification. Each channel is responsible for eliminating or detoxifying toxic material that can harm the inside and outside of your body. These channels are:

- The Liver
- The Lungs
- The Lymphatic System
- The Colon
- Kidneys
- Skin
- Blood

The Liver

Your liver is responsible for detoxifying all your body's blood as it comes from your intestines, colon, lungs, and lymphatic system. Once detoxified, this blood moves into your entire body, to provide your cells with oxygen and nutrients.

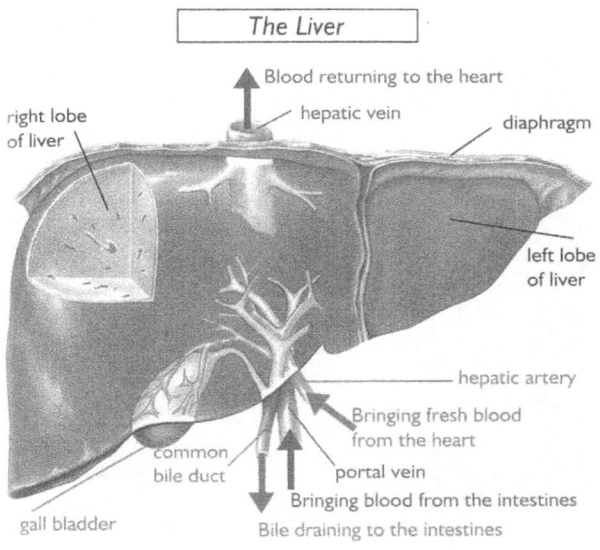

Because you drink, eat and breathe in so many toxins, your liver has a hard time neutralizing all of them. If you are constipated, this puts an extreme toxic load on your liver. The liver will eventually route some of these toxins to your skin and face.

All cellular wastes are routed to your liver, through your lymphatic system. Excess hormones come to your liver from the blood. Once cellular waste and hormones are in the liver, it starts the detoxifying process. If your liver is overloaded with toxins, it will start to store these toxins in its own cells, in your other organs, in your joints, in your fatty tissue, in your skin, or any other place that it can find.

Hormones, such as androgens, that are not neutralized can get back into your blood stream and move into your facial follicles. In your follicle, these hormones pile up and cause an over production of sebum.

If you are a typical eater, most likely, you have been living on poor-quality food and eating a lot of junk food. This food contains toxic chemicals that will accumulate in your colon, your liver, your blood, your tissue, and in your skin. These toxins need to be neutralized and eliminated by your seven elimination channels.

The Lungs

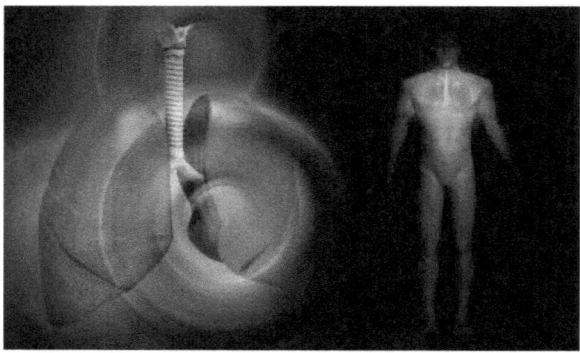

You have two large sacs that are called lungs. As you breathe in air, your blood pulls oxygen out of this air, which is routed to your liver. Then, your blood moves this oxygen into your heart and to all parts of your body.

As you breathe out, waste and carbon dioxide are pushed out through your mouth.

Your cells use oxygen to create energy, for your body. You need energy for every movement you make. Oxygen is also used to neutralize waste and pathogens. The more acid waste and pathogens you have, the more oxygen is used up, to neutralize them. This means you will have less oxygen for other necessary body functions.

If your other elimination channels are weak and overloaded with waste, your lungs will also become overloaded, trying to get rid of this waste. This will weaken your lungs.

The result of weak lungs is that more waste stays in your body, making it more acidic and susceptible to disease and infections. As your body gets more toxic, so does your blood. This toxic matter can eventually reach your facial follicles and feed the bad bacteria that are there.

The Lymphatic System

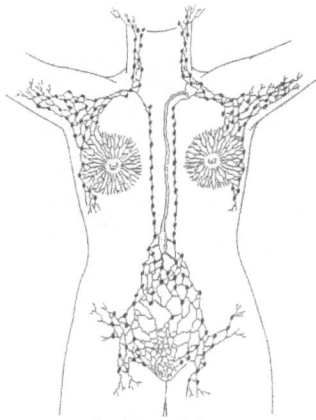

Your lymphatic system is part of your immune system. It consists of a series of tubes, large and small, that cover your entire body. Through these tubes flow whitish liquid called lymph. Since this system does not have a pump, your lymph is pushed through the tubes by your body's movement.

Lymph liquid surrounds all your body cells and is responsible for bringing nutrients from your blood to your cells. As your cells excrete waste into your lymph, the lymph moves this waste into your lymphatic tubes. Your lymph liquid travels up these tubes to lymph nodes that detoxify it and then send it back into your blood stream.

Toxins and pathogens that are in your lymph liquid are moved into lymph nodes. In your lymph nodes, this toxic matter is neutralized into harmless chemicals and then moved into your liver for elimination.

Your lymph liquid is composed of electrolyte minerals such as sodium, potassium, calcium, phosphorus, and chloride. So, strong lymph liquid is built when you eat fruits and vegetables.

Excess toxic waste accumulates in your lymph liquid, when your body does not have enough electrolyte minerals to neutralize them. When your lymph nodes become overwhelmed with toxic waste from your cells and blood, they become inflamed and cannot keep your body free of toxic matter. Now, your body is considered acidic, and you will have a difficult time fighting infections, such as acne.

The Colon

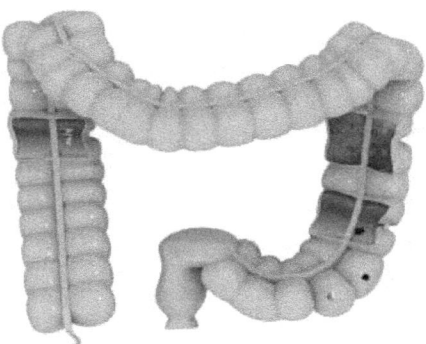

Your colon is where most illnesses or diseases start, and this includes your acne.
Your colon collects toxins, pathogens, and acid waste. If you have constipation, these toxins and acid waste can penetrate your colon walls

and get reabsorbed into your blood. When waste gets back into your blood, some of it can be routed to your facial follicles, causing skin inflammation or pimples. This is the waste that you need to make sure does not reach your facial follicles.

The first thing you want to know about your colon is whether you are constipated.

If you are constipated, your colon has a lot of functions that it can't perform properly. When your fecal matter reaches your colon, it is already toxic. If it stays in your colon for more than a day, it becomes even more toxic.

Constipation causes this toxic matter to be reabsorbed back into your blood stream and back to your liver. When your liver is overloaded with toxins, some of these toxins are not neutralized, by the liver, and escape into your blood.

Most people are constipated. It is typical for people to go 2-3 days without a bowel movement. Some doctors say it's acceptable or normal for this to happen. **This is not acceptable.** If you want to become seriously ill, or if you want to struggle with acne for a long time, then it might be ok. Fecal matter that stays in your colon, more than normal, starts to,

- affect the health of your colon
- cause colon wall inflammation
- decay and become toxic
- harden on colon walls
- interfere with absorption of nutrients
- kill good bacteria that keeps you healthy
- promote multiplication of bad bacteria
- stick to your colon walls
- weaken your colon walls

When you have constipation, this means that fecal matter,
- moves slowly in the colon
- becomes stagnant and doesn't move for days
- moves out the anus, but some of it sticks to the colon walls
- has a hard time coming out

So what can you do about constipation? You will get a plan for this, in a later chapter.

The kidneys

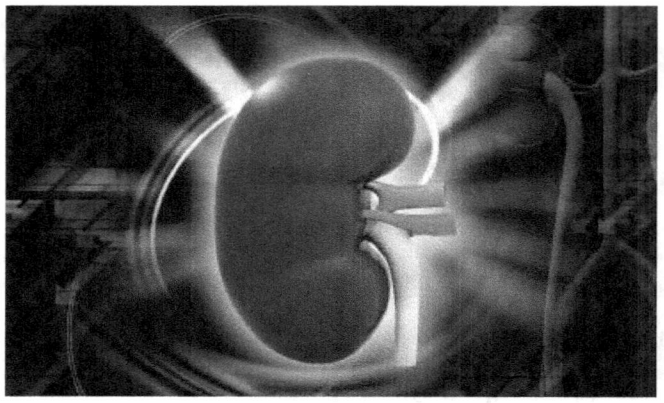

The purpose of your kidneys is to filter your blood. About four gallons of water are filtered every day from your blood, but only around three pints are pulled out as urine.

Alcohol and sugar are the most damaging to your kidneys, since they kill kidney cells and weaken your kidneys' function.

Drinking plenty of water is one way to keep waste from accumulating in your body. You need to drink plenty of water daily, so your kidneys can remove toxins and excess nutrients, vitamins, and minerals from your blood.

When you drink plenty of water, your skin does not have to act as a filter to remove excess waste from your blood, since it will be excreted as urine, by your kidney.

Water also is needed to keep your skin moist. Water in your skin layers helps to protect your skin from bacteria and toxins that try to pass into your skin.

The more fresh juices you drink and the more fruits or vegetables you eat, the less water you need to drink. All juices contain plenty of distilled water, which contributes to your daily water requirements.

Drinking sodas and other drinks that have sugar cannot be

counted as water.

The Skin

Your skin is the largest of the elimination channels. Your blood feeds your follicles, but also brings toxins, acid wastes, and hormones to them. It is this waste that has to be eliminated through your skin.

If you are frequently constipated, then your liver will be overworked and unable to detoxify all your colon toxins. Your liver has to detoxify all the toxic matter that comes from the food you eat and the air you breathe.

However, when you have excessive body toxins, they get into your skin follicles where they cause inflammation and plugged pores. In many cases, these toxins reach your skin surface, through sweat, causing body odor.

If your skin, throughout your body, is clean and its pores are open and unclogged, a normal level of toxins will move out through your pores without creating pimples or eruptions. Your skin normally moves 1-2 pounds of toxins out of your skin daily.

To keep your skin active and serving as a good channel of elimination, you need to brush your skin daily, before you shower or during your shower.

In her book, Detox For Life, 2002, Loree Taylor Jordan, C.C.H., I.D. says,

"One of greatest gifts of health that you can give yourself is the gift of skin brushing. Dry skin brushing is one of the finest of all baths. No soap can wash the skin as clean as the new skin you have under the old. You make new skin on your body every 24 hours. The skin will only be as clean as the bloodstream. Dry skin brushing removes the top layer. This helps to eliminate uric acid crystals, catarrh, and various other acids in the body. The skin should eliminate 2 pounds of waste acids daily."

The Blood

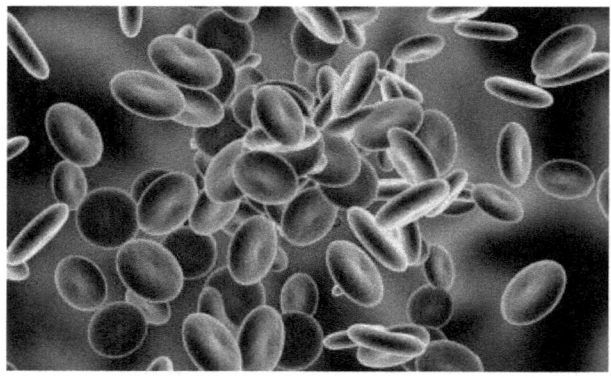

Your blood is considered a liquid organ. As such, it acts to assist the elimination channels to get rid of wastes. Blood is delivered from all parts of your body back to your liver to get detoxified and purified. Blood is also routed to your kidneys where your blood pH is maintained, and various nutrients are reused and others are eliminated through urine.

Your lymph liquid is also routed back into your blood, purified by your lymph nodes and liver, and returned to your lymph system.

Your blood travels in and out of your lungs to eliminate carbon dioxide and to get oxygen, which is delivered to your cells and organs.

Blood is the work horse that moves toxic waste out of your body and moves in oxygen and nutrients into your cells and tissues. Keeping your blood clean is critical for eliminating acne. When your blood is over loaded with toxins, they get into your facial pores and plug them up.

Other Avenues of Acid Creation

There are four other important areas that you need to know about that contribute to acid waste. If these areas are not working properly, then acid waste is created.

- Stomach acid

- Thyroid

- Pancreatic digestive enzymes

- Attitude

Stomach Acid

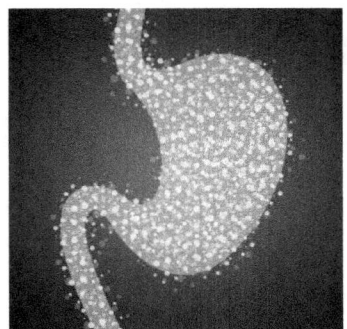

Your stomach uses Hydrochloric acid (HCl) to break down protein. It also has many other functions, such as,

- killing pathogens and microbes

- controlling the adsorption of most B-complex vitamins.

- controlling the adsorption of iron, calcium, zinc, copper, magnesium.

- controlling the adsorption of vitamin C

- maintaining the correct pH for good digestion

- preventing constipation

When you have low levels of HCl stomach acid, chances are that you will be susceptible to getting acne. Low HCL levels do not allow you to digest your food properly, causing undigested food to reach your colon, where it becomes toxic.

The Thyroid

Your thyroid function plays an important role in your health and in acne.

If you have an underactive thyroid, the symptoms associated with this condition are weight gain, fatigue, lack of energy, lack of patience, trouble concentrating, constipation, dry skin, thinning hair, feeling cold, high cholesterol, or restlessness. These symptoms can lead to depression, arguments, anxiety, or loss of sex drive. Other symptoms may include,

- Memory loss
- Cold hands or feet
- Inability to lose weight
- Menstrual problems
- Migraines
- Hypertension
- Infertility

If you have an overactive thyroid, some symptoms are nervousness, anxiety, insomnia, racing heartbeat, excess perspiration or weight loss. These symptoms can lead to other psychological issues.

You will be testing yourself for low or high thyroid function, in chapter 12. All the diets and cleansing in this program, will help you stabilize your thyroid. You will be able to test for thyroid function at different times in this program, so that you can gauge your thyroid health.

Pancreatic Digestive Enzymes

When the food you eat passes your stomach and enters your

small intestine, your pancreas releases digestive enzymes and bicarbonate to help complete your digestive process.

The bicarbonate helps to neutralize the acid food that comes from your stomach. Your digestive enzymes digest carbohydrates, fats, and protein that were not digested in your stomach.

When your pancreas loses its efficiency and releases fewer digestive enzymes, less food is properly digested. This results in more undigested food reaching your colon. When this happens, your undigested food, if it stays too long in your colon, becomes a source of rotting matter and toxic material.
A healthy pancreas provides the digestive juices to digest the food you eat. This prevents acne and other skin eruptions to occur.

This program calls for taking digestive enzyme capsules to help you digest your food better. When you take these enzymes and eat more fruit and vegetables, you take a load off your pancreas, giving it time to rebuild itself.

Your Attitude

The way you think and act is also expressed in your skin. Since your brain is not separate from your physical well-being, distorted thoughts and feelings can cause illness and disease.
Negative thoughts and feeling are known to produce chemicals that are toxic. These toxic chemicals need to be eliminated through the elimination channels.

Toxic thoughts and feelings are typically eliminated through an eighth channel of elimination called the "channel of behavior." Toxic thoughts are released by various bad behaviors, attitudes, addictions and act outs.

Acne can be related to your emotion of fear or anxiety. It can also be an expression of holding onto to old traumatic or unpleasant memories. Acne can be a way of burying traumatic or toxic memories into your skin. It is these memories that are trying to surface, but you may not be ready to know what they are, so you hold on to them through acne.

Reducing your anxiety, fear, or anger is also part of becoming a healthier person. This is an area that you need to work on, so that you can eventually become cured of acne. **Chapter 21** has more information on how to reduce stress.

Outline of the Acne Program

Here is an outline of the various processes you need to follow.

A step by step program will be given to you at the end of this book.

- health Tests
- constipation diet
- body cleansing
- facial cleansing
- kidney cleansing
- liver cleansing and diet
- body cycle diet
- mediating
- exercising
- herbal drinks and tonics to drink
- supplements for immunity

Controlling Acne

Because acne is a combination of many different factors, the cure for acne must be approached aggressively, from many different fronts. This is what this acne program does. In the following chapters, you will find aggressive approaches for each factor that creates acne.

Chapter Summary

Acne occurs when your elimination channels are not processing toxins and hormones the way they should. When these toxins and hormones reach your facial follicles, they start a chemical cascade that results in plugged follicles and acne.

Excess sebum production occurs when your hormones are out of balance. This causes follicles to become plugged. Bacteria favor blocked follicles and they starts to multiple, which ends up infecting and inflaming your follicles.

Polycystic ovary syndrome (PCOS) affects many women. In this syndrome, the ovaries malfunction causing inability to ovulate. High levels of male hormones typically exist in women with PCOS. Women with this condition tend to have acne, because of hormonal imbalances.

High insulin levels are associated with acne. It will be important to control sugar levels, to keep acne under control.

You have **Seven Channels of Elimination** to remove physical toxins from your body and **One Channel** to remove negative thoughts and stress. All of these channels must be working properly, so that excess toxins are not excreted through your skin. These channels are brought back into balance through cleansing, diet and supplementation.

Digestion is critical in maintaining the health of your channels of elimination. It is your stomach that digests your food and provides you with the nutrients that give you health.

Without the proper digestive enzymes in your stomach and small intestine, you will create colon toxins that appear in your skin.

Without good **Thyroid Function**, you will be susceptible to acne. Without good metabolism at your cell level, you will not create the nutrients you need to keep your elimination channels healthy. These channels will be overwhelmed with acid waste and cause your blood and body to become toxic.

Chapter 5: Candida And Parasites Elimination

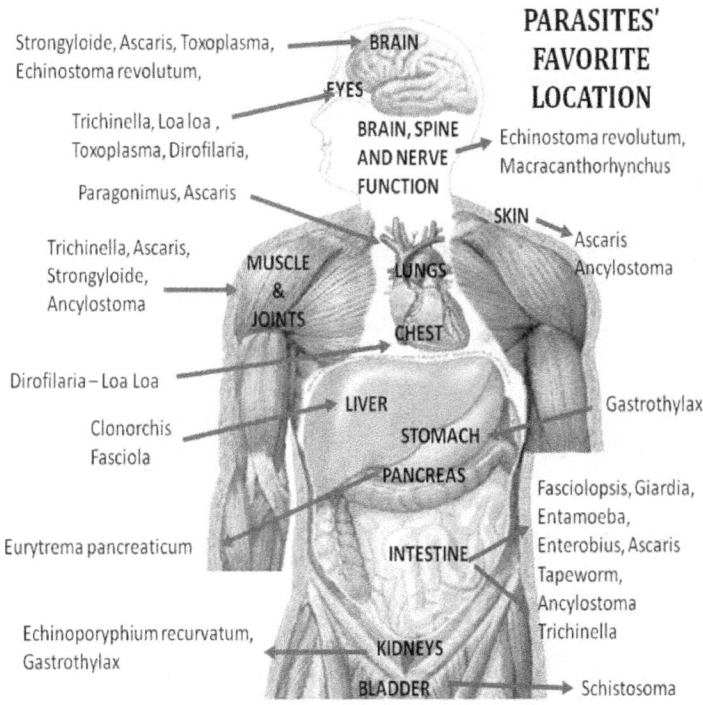

PARASITES' FAVORITE LOCATION

Strongyloide, Ascaris, Toxoplasma, Echinostoma revolutum, — BRAIN

EYES

Trichinella, Loa loa, Toxoplasma, Dirofilaria, — BRAIN, SPINE AND NERVE FUNCTION

Echinostoma revolutum, Macracanthorhynchus

Paragonimus, Ascaris

SKIN — Ascaris, Ancylostoma

Trichinella, Ascaris, Strongyloide, Ancylostoma — MUSCLE & JOINTS LUNGS CHEST

Dirofilaria – Loa Loa

LIVER

Gastrothylax

Clonorchis Fasciola

STOMACH PANCREAS

Eurytrema pancreaticum

INTESTINE

Fasciolopsis, Giardia, Entamoeba, Enterobius, Ascaris Tapeworm, Ancylostoma Trichinella

Echinoporyphium recurvatum, Gastrothylax

KIDNEYS

BLADDER — Schistosoma

Parasites in Your Body

Parasites are everywhere, and their eggs are found in all areas where you walk, live, play, touch, swim, and travel. They even appear in some water supplies. They live on or in humans, animals, and plants.

Most people have some parasites and don't even know it.

Flukes and Worms

There are hundreds of flat round worm species. Liver flukes

are the most common parasite in the USA. These worms and flukes live in your colon, liver, and throughout your body, reducing your health. Flukes are difficult to avoid, no matter how clean you are, since they are found throughout the world on food, silverware, glasses, air, water, napkins.

If you have flukes, your symptoms might be fatigue, craving for fat, slight dark skin tone, and a sad appearance on your face.

Candida Albicans and Fungi

Candida albicans and fungi are also parasites. They are hardy and are found throughout your body. If you have Candida, you may have gas, bloating, confusion, weight gain, brain fog, and many other symptoms.

Candida is a yeast-like organism, which is found in your mouth, throat, intestines and vagina. Candida always exists in your body, but it's kept under control by your good bacteria. However, when your diet is poor, your body becomes inflamed and Candida multiples. If you use antibiotics, drugs, steroids, or contraceptive pills, Candida will also flourish.

When Candida has control of your colon, it becomes an overactive fermentation tube, where excess gas, bloating, and irregular bowels occur.

If Candida grows tendrils, these tendrils can penetrate your large intestine walls and spread toxins into your blood. This blood does not pass through your liver, which would detoxify it, but gets into your body, causing allergies, fatigue, and untraceable illnesses.

Eliminating Parasites

Making your body more alkaline will help you minimize or eliminate parasites. It takes time to make your body alkaline, but, you can do by eating specific fruits and vegetables. The transformation of changing your acid body into an alkaline body can take up to a year or more. So little by little you can make your body alkaline, if you eat the right food.

Parasite feed on sugars, fruit fructose, fats, and oils. If you eat less of this food, you will reduce the parasites that live in your body.

Just assume you have parasites, since there are no tests that can detect all the parasites you might have. The best you can do is to reduce the quantity and the variety of parasites that you have.

The best way to get rid of parasites is to make your body uncomfortable for them to live in. To do this, you need to have an alkaline body, bring in more oxygen into your blood, change your diet, and drink specific herbal remedies.

Herbal Remedies

The herbal remedies that are effective in killing parasites are:
- Wormwood
- Black walnut
- Cloves
- Oregano oil
- Grapefruit seed extract
- Garlic

You can get herbal extracts of wormwood, black walnut, oregano oil, and grapefruit seed extract. These are the best herbals to use to get rid of parasites and Candida.

Diet Changes

Certain diet changes are necessary to minimize the population of parasites and bad bacteria. Avoid eating sweets and sugars, fructose, starches, grains, and some fruits, milk, and fat. All of these foods provide nutrients for bacteria, causing them to multiply.

How to Tell If You Have Yeast or Parasites

There are many symptoms that are associated with having parasites. If you have a few of these, you might have parasites. However, this list is in no way an absolute indication that you have   Candida.

Symptoms of Yeast and Parasite Overgrowth
- Lowered immune system and constant illness
- Rectal itching, especially at night
- More than one vaginal yeast infection
- Sores on your mouth or lips or white spots inside your mouth
- Difficulty sleeping and waking up
- Toe fungus or athletes foot
- Bloating and gas
- Sensitivity to food or chemicals
- Sensitivity to the smell of strong perfumes or cigarette smoke
- Rashes or itching around genitals in men or women
- Recurrent bladder infections
- Food cravings, especially for sweet or starchy foods
- History of antibiotic or steroid use
- History of contraceptive use

- Brain fog or mental fuzziness
- Menstrual irregularities, including irregular periods, heavy bleeding, cramps, PMS, or anovulation
- Anxiety or depression
- Constipation or diarrhea
- History of eating high sugar/carbohydrate foods

Getting Rid of Parasites

It will be important to get rid parasites, since they suppress your immune system and create an imbalance, in your hormones. In the following chapters, you will discover how to eliminate parasites.

Chapter Summary

Here are the main points from this chapter.

You can get parasites from all public places. When these parasites and bacteria invade your body, they can establish a home in any part of your body. Just assume you have parasites. Everyone has them.

Candida is one of the most infectious and insidious bacteria that create body damage. The best way to minimize or eliminate parasites and Candida is to make it uncomfortable for them to live in your body. The best way to do this is to make your body alkaline, by changing your diet and by drinking special herbal teas that kill them.

When you **have parasites**, you can have an array of symptoms. The list of symptoms provided in this chapter will help you to identify possible signs of parasites in your body. However, having a few or many of these symptoms is not confirmation of having parasites. Just assume you have them.

Herbal teas help to eliminate and control parasites. Using herbs like oregano oil, garlic, and wormwood are excellent ways of eliminate parasites.

Parasites lower your immune system. They produce toxic excretions that need to be eliminated. They thrive in an acid body and use sugar and simple carbohydrates as their food. They affect your liver function. To be acne free, you need to eliminate or reduce them to a point where they have no effect in your body.

Chapter 6: Acne - Essential Fatty Acids

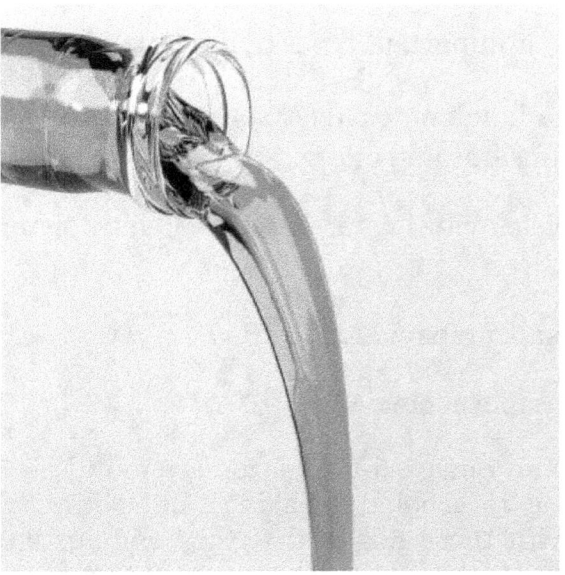

Essential Fatty Acids

Essential fatty acids are the omega-3 and omega-6. These omegas break down into other essential fatty acids that are found in fish oil. You can find omegas, in certain amounts, in most of the oils that you purchase in health food and regular grocery stores. These omegas are called essential, because you cannot create them in your body, and your cells need and use them every day.

If you do not eat enough of these essential fatty acids, you're going to get sick. It's a good idea not to be short on essential fatty acids.

Most people eat around 15 tablespoons of Omega-6 to one tablespoon of **Omega-3**. If you are one of these persons, then you can expect to come down with any of the inflammatory diseases, like arthritis, arteriosclerosis, colitis, eczema, ulcers, or acne.

What are Essential Fatty Acids?

There are four important types of Essential Fatty Acids:

- Alpha Linolenic Acid (ALA) or **Omega-3** Oil, a polyunsaturated oil

- Linoleic Acid (LA) or Omega-6 Oil, a polyunsaturated oil

- Eicosapentaenoic Acid (EPA)

- Docosahexaenoic Acid (DHA)

Omega-3 and omega-6 fatty acids are found in everyday oils that you use for cooking, baking, and eating. One of the problems with these oils is that they contain more omega-6 than **omega-3.** And, it is the **omega-3** that most people lack in their diet.

Oils that Contain Omegas

Flax seed oil – contains four times more **omega-3** than omega-6. For this reason, flax seeds and its oil have become popular. However, as you will see later, your body may not be able to break down flax seed oil into the needed EPA and DHA fatty acids.

Perilla seed oil – contains three to four times more **omega-3** than omega-6. For this reason, this is an excellent oil to use, but is not very popular.

Hemp oil – contains the ideal ratio of 4:1, four times more omega-6 than **omega-3.** Since it is derived from the marijuana plant, it does not have a good image. But, you can still get it online and many people are using it. You should eat 3 to 4 times more omega-6 than omega-3.

Pumpkin oil–contains three times more omega-6 than **omega-3**.
Walnut oil-contains ten times more omega-6 than **omega-3.**

Safflower – has no omega-3, and 75% of its oil is omega-6
Sunflower–has no omega-3 and 65% of its oil is omega-6. This is not a good oil to use to get the omegas, unless you use it with oil that is high in **omega-3**

Wheat germ oil–has slight amounts of omega-3 but is mostly omega-6

Olive oil–has very little omega-3 and 8% of its oil is omega-6

Corn oil–contains mostly omega-6

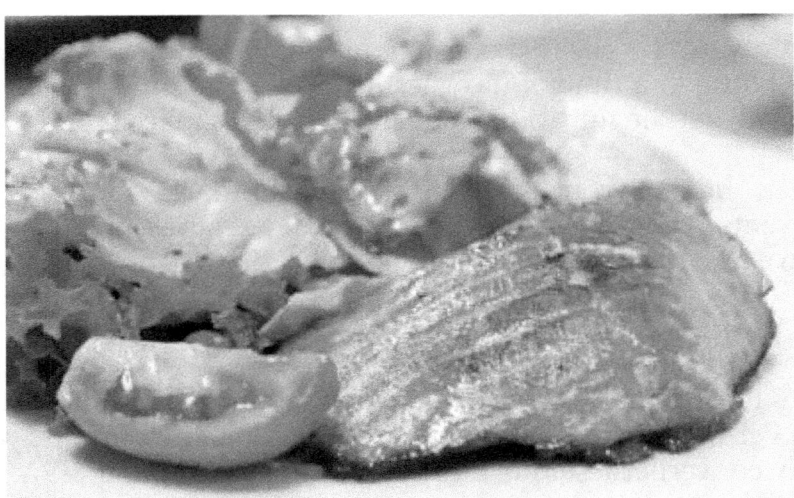

You can see that most oils have very little omega-3, and this is why people use flax seeds and its oil in their salads.

Fish Oils

Fish are high in EPA and DHA fatty acid oils. Include fish in your diet, by eating it at least one or twice a week. Your body breaks down omega oils into EPA and DHA fatty acids. But, by eating fish, which has natural EPA and DHA, you bypass the body's process of converting omegas into EPA and DHA.

The fish to eat are,

- Salmon
- Sardines
- Halibut
- Trout
- Albacore tuna
- Mackerel

Buying Oils

When you use oils, it is best to alternate between oils, using one bottle at a time of flax, perilla, and hemp oil. In this way, you will get the nutritional benefits that the different oils.

When buying your oils, buy them in dark bottles. This prevents oxidation from occurring, and assures that you get active and fresh oils that contain strong levels of omegas.

EPA and DHA in Fish Oil

EPA and DHA are also considered essential fatty acids. When you eat flax seed oil or any oil that contains the omegas, your body converts these oils into EPA and DHA. It is the EPA and DHA that your body needs.

To do this conversion, your body needs is a little help from enzymes called,

- Delta-5 desaturase
- Delta-6 desaturase

It is these enzymes that convert omega-3 and omega-6 into useful and necessary fatty acids – EPA, DHA, GLA, DGLA.
But, these enzymes also need help from zinc, magnesium, vitamin B6, and biotin to make the final conversion.

EPA and DHA in Fish Oil?

Fish oil contains EPA and DHA , so you can save your body the trouble of making them from omega-3 and omega-6. In fact, this might be a good idea, since your body may not be able to make EPA and DHA from the omegas.

Why would your body not be converting the Omega-3 or Omega-6 oils to the much-needed DHA and EPA fatty oils? There are quite a few reasons for this. Certain diets and body conditions block your conversion of omegas into the needed DHA and EPA, such as,

- Aging reducing the power of desaturase 5 & 6 enzyme
- Being exposed to excess stress, anxiety, or fear
- Drinking too much caffeine or alcohol & smoking
- absorbing excess toxins from the air, water and food
- Eating too much hydrogenated or partially hydrogenated oils that contain
  trans-fatty acids.
- Eating too many refined carbohydrates
- Eating too much saturated fat from milk, butter, beef
- Eating too much sugar or being overweight
- Having a zinc deficiency

- Having cancer, diabetes or eczema caused by allergies
- Having frequent viral infections
- Lacking the sufficient desaturase enzymes
- Not eating a balance of omega-3 or 6 oils
- Using pharmaceutical drugs or NASID's aspirin)

As you can see, it is not enough to add more omegas into your diet, if you have an unhealthy way of eating and living. A poor lifestyle will destroy or block the use of essential fatty acids in your body. You can now see why so many people become sick as they age. They lack the omegas.

Because the omega oils, EPA, and DHA, each have certain chemical activities in your body, it is important to supplement with these oils.

So what are GLA and DGLA?

Gamma-Linolenic acid or GLA is an omega-6 fatty acid.

GLA needs to be chemically created in your body. Your body takes omega-6 and converts it to GLA, using the Delta-5 or 6 desaturase enzyme.

Now, **DGLA** stands for Dihomo-gamma-Linolenic Acid. As you will see later EPA, DHA, and DGLA will continue to be broken down or changed into other fatty acids that your body will eventually use to protect itself from disease, including acne.

A lot of GLA that is created from omega 6 is converted to the nutrient called DGLA that fights inflammation. Having enough magnesium, zinc, vitamins C, B3, and B6 in your body will help change GLA to DGLA.

The Breakdown of Fatty Acids in Your Body

Let's follow the path of the chemical changes of omega oils in your body. Let's see what function they have in your body and why they are so critical for your health.

Let's start with omega-3.

Omega-3

The Delta-6 desaturase enzymes (that we mentioned above) break down omega-3 first into,

Stearidonic Acid

Then the delta-5 desaturase enzyme breaks down Stearidonic Acid into EPA (Eicosapentaenoic acid.)

EPA is then changed into DHA (Docosahexaenoic Acid) by the delta-6 desaturase. So, omega-3 is changed into EPA and DHA.

It is important to know that omega-3 is changed into EPA and DHA in your body. You can bypass this process, if you use fish oil, since fish oil already consists of EPA and DHA.
Now, EPA and DHA are further broken down into other chemicals. Now we're getting into those chemicals that work at the cellular level, which are called **"prostaglandins."**

This is how this happens:

EPA creates series 1 prostaglandins (PGE1)
DHA creates series 3 prostaglandins (PGE3)
Eicosapentaenoic Acid (EPA)

Because EPA is a long-chain fatty acid, it is more susceptible to attack from free radicals in your body. So it has a short life cycle. This means that you need to eat more omega-3 oil every day or take a good EPA supplement to maintain a good supply of omega-3 in your blood.

EPA is important for your body because it creates prostaglandins. In addition, EPA and DHA form the structure of cells walls. They are necessary in the function and development of your brain, eyes, and skin.

Docosahexaenoic Acid (DHA)

You can now see that Omega-3 oils can break down into EPA and DHA. This breakdown process, in your body, is slow and complex. In some cases, certain people are not able to produce EPA and DHA from omega-3, because they produce defective delta-6 desaturase enzymes.

This creates a real health problem, if you can't produce EPA and DHA from the Omega-3. But there is a way around this.

So, how do you know, if you are not breaking down omega-3 to produce EPA and DHA? There is no easy way to tell except through blood tests, or if you have specific illnesses that point to this breakdown. Just to be on the safe side, it is best to supplement your diet with fish oil capsules, which consist of EPA and DHA.

Make sure you use a fish oil supplement that contains vitamin E to protect the oil from oxidation.

Omega-6 chemically changes

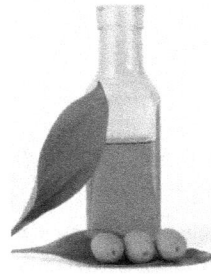

It's the Delta-6 desaturase enzymes and specific vitamins with zinc that breakdown omega-6 first into,

- Gamma-Linolenic Acid (GLA)

- Then this changes into,

- Dihomo-gamma-linolenic   acid

(DGLA)

- Then into,
- Arachidonic Acid (AA)
- And finally, AA can change into,
- Docospentaenoic acid (DPA)

DPA is not found in fish oils and only in the omegas. It is a highly important fatty acid and
is found in high concentrations in your blood. It is found in harp seals, which have a high concentration of Omega-3 and is the secret of Eskimo health, since they eat a lot of seals.

Both Omega-3 and Omega-6 can chemically change to create some DPA. DPA is not available through flax seed oil or other plant based oils.

Some products, such as Gold Omega-3 seal oil, give you plenty of DPA.

Where do all of these chemical changes lead to?

They lead to more prostaglandins.

Dihomo-gamma-linolenic acid **(DGLA)** creates series 1 prostaglandins (PGE1)

Arachidonic Acid (AA) creates series 2 prostaglandins (PGE2)
Fish-Oil Capsules

When supplementing with fish-oil capsules, make sure the product contains both the EPA and DHA. These fatty acids work together in providing the benefits and activities necessary for good health.

Fatty Acid Deficiency

When you are deficient in the essential fatty acids, you will have,

- a weaken immune system
- inflammatory disorders
- poor skin
- skin eruptions and other wounds that won't heal
- sebum production increases
- sebaceous glands that increase in size

Eating essential oils is necessary to provide the right oils that are used in the sebaceous glands. These oils can come from straight vegetable oils or from oils in specific foods such as nuts and seeds.

Chapter Summary

The essential fatty acids, omega-3 and 6 are necessary, if you want to eliminate your acne. Eating the right food and supplementing
with flax seed and fish oil are one of the best ways to use these fatty acids.

There are many oils that you can use in your salad or food to get omega-3 and 6. Your body needs more 3 times more omega-6 than omega-3, and certain oils can provide this.

Eating fish is a great idea for getting more omegas into your diet. A good fish oil supplement is the recommend way to get the omegas.

Fish-oil supplements have EPA and DHA that your body needs. EPA and DHA are reduced in your body into prostaglandin.

Without the proper amount of the omega oils in your diet, you will develop terminal diseases. These oils are also instrumental in keeping your hormones in balance and preventing your follicles from becoming contaminated and inflamed.

Chapter 7: Starting Your Acne Cure Program

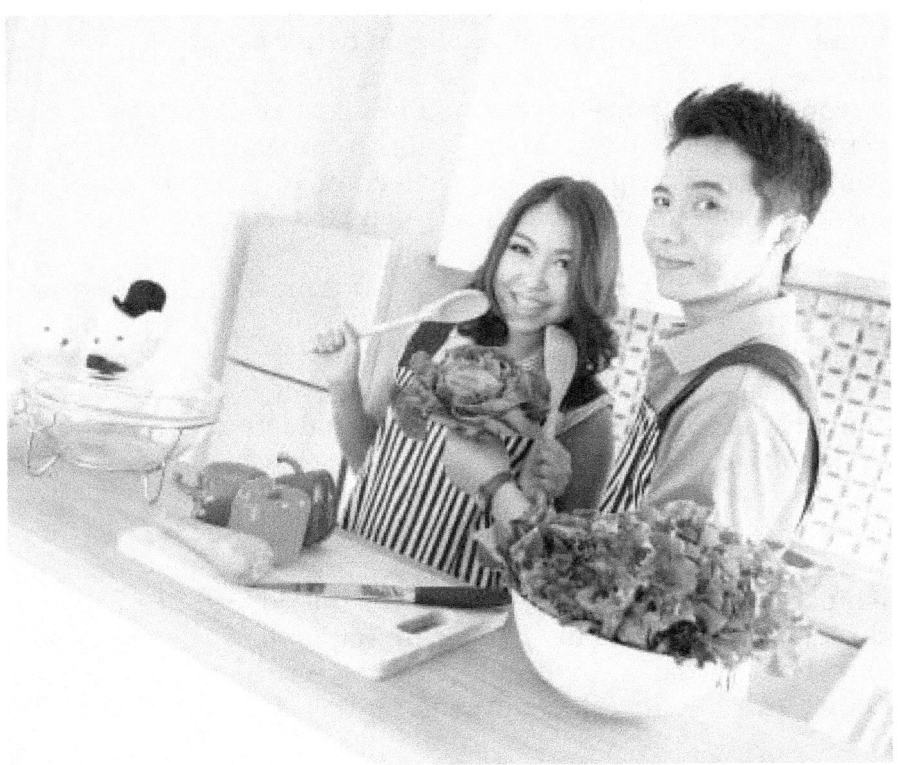

The Acne Cure

Here is the start of your acne program. Each chapter that follows is one step that you need to complete in some manner. These chapters are not listed in the order you need to follow. The final chapter will give a step by step program to follow, which includes information from the various chapters.

Since acne is an imbalanced condition that occurs from within your body, it tends to exhibits this imbalance on your face. So you need to:

- attack the problem from inside your body

- attack the problem from outside your body

If your acne is not too severe, you may not need to do all the steps in this program. However, try to do each step, since not only is this program about acne, but it's about improving your immune system, so that you can gain better health.

If your acne is more severe, follow most of the steps in this acne program. Remember, acne is an expression of your whole-body system and is a reflection of what is going on inside your mind, cell structure and internal organs.

You will be doing a lot of cleansing, but most of this cleansing comes from changing your diet and drinking more fruit and vegetable juices
and herbal tonics. Your kidney and liver cleanse are more complex and it's better to buy these products that are already designed for these cleanses.

Acne is an excessive toxic condition within your body, where your elimination channels have become sluggish. When his happens, your toxins move into your blood and are excreted through your skin. This is an automatic survival mechanism your body initiates, in an effort to protect the insides of your body – cells, liquid, blood, organs, and tissue.

Starting the Acne Program Steps

If you follow this program, it will not only cure your acne, but it will provide you with a nutritional program that can become part of your lifestyle.

Here are the areas that cover this program. These areas will be outlined in the 10-week program plan.

1. Eliminating Constipation
2. Body Cleansing
3. Kidney Cleansing

4. Liver Cleansing

5. Stress Relief & Sleep

6. Changing Attitude

7. Herbal Remedies for Acne

8. Supplements for Acne

9. Supplementing with Essential Fatty Acids

10. First Facial Cleansing

11. Second Facial Cleansing

12. Third Facial Cleansing

13. A Diet for Acne

14. Natural Way to Eat

15. Sunshine, Air, and Water

16. Brushing Your Skin

17. Acne Program Summary Step by Step

Chapter Summary

Here are the main points from this chapter. These are the key ideas that you will be using when you start this program.

Now you are almost ready to start your acne program.

In this program, you will be using natural health techniques to cleanse your body, improve your regularity, strengthen your elimination organs, balance your hormones, and cleansing your skin.

The main purpose of this program is to eliminate an overload of toxins within your body that have caused your body to malfunction. This malfunction is reflected on your facial skin, as acne.

There are **17 different areas** that you need to go through to complete this acne program. When you finish this program, you will find a few new diets that will help you maintain an acne-free body.

Chapter 8: Constipation Transit Time

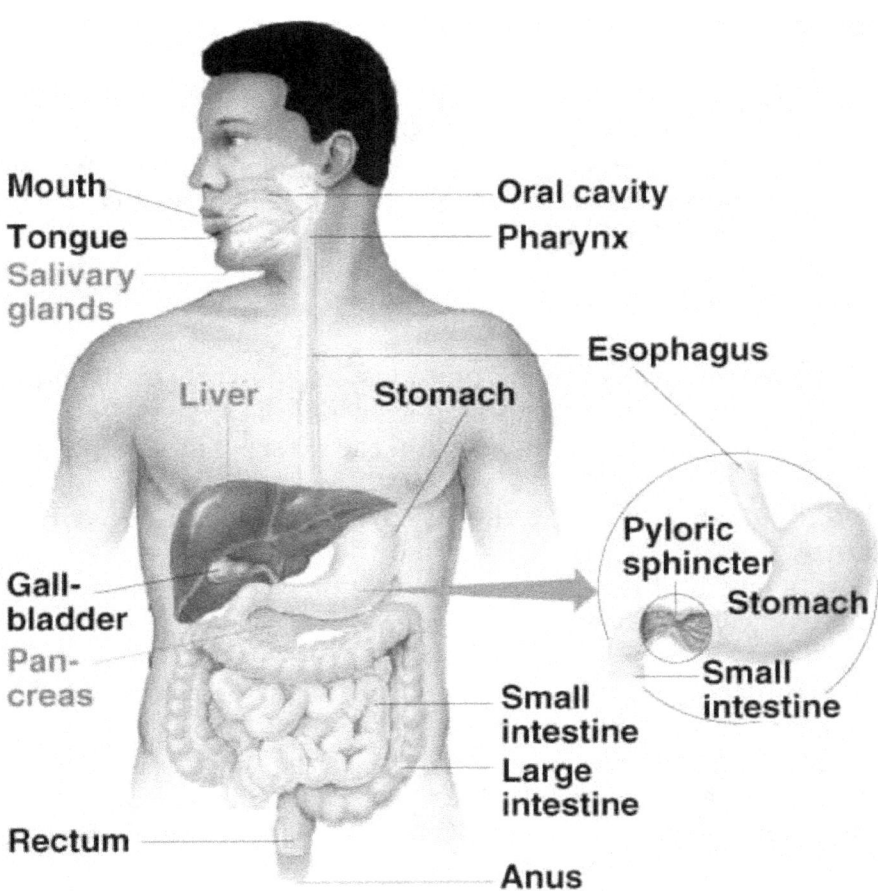

Mouth

Tongue

Salivary glands

Oral cavity

Pharynx

Esophagus

Liver

Stomach

Gall-bladder

Pan-creas

Pyloric sphincter

Stomach

Small intestine

Small intestine

Large intestine

Rectum

Anus

Transit Time Test

Here is a test called "Transit Time" that you can use to determine how long it takes for your food to travel through your intestinal tract. This test measures the time it takes food to be digested as it travels from your mouth to your anus and expelled as a stool.

Medical Transient Time

Doctors can test your transit time by having you take a marker pill that shows its position in x-rays, as it travels through your digestive system. The test that you will do here is not that precise.

This test is just to give you an idea on whether your transit time is short or long. Your transit time varies on what type of food you eat and the amount of fiber and water it has. Protein and whole grains take longer to digest, whereas fruits, vegetables and juices take less.

Ideal Transient Time

There are many different opinions as to what is the ideal transit time. Transit times from 8 to 14 hours, 12 to 18 hours, and 33 to 47 hours are reported on the Internet as good times.

It's best to have a transit time of around 16 to 22 hours or so.
This means that if you have 3 meals a day, you will have two to three bowel movements per day.

One thing to be aware of is, if you have one or two bowel movements per day, you may still be constipated. This can happen, if the bowel movements, you are having are coming from food eaten three to four days ago. This is why it is important to test your transit time, to make sure your digested food is not staying more than a day in your colon.

When you have a transit time of 48 hours or longer, you increase your risk of cancer, diverticulitis, and overgrowth of Candida. You also start the re-absorption of toxic colon matter back into your blood stream.

Start Testing Transit Time

There are a few ways to check your transit time. What you want to do is drink a colored drink that has the properties of a natural dye. You can use chlorophyll liquid, the juice of red beets or active charcoal. Or, you can eat only corn as a meal and then wait to see how long it takes to shows up in your stools.

Here's how to start. Right after a meal, drink a glass of chlorophyll or red beet juice.

Preparing Your Chlorophyll Drink

- Add 1-2 oz. of liquid chlorophyll into an empty glass
- Squeeze the juice from one lemon into the glass
- Fill the glass with 8 oz. of distilled water
- Drink the combination completely

Chlorophyll has a dull and blank taste. By adding lemon juice to the chlorophyll drink, you make it more palatable. Drink this drink right after a meal.

Red Beet Juice

You can buy some red beet juice or you can take some beets and put them through your juicer. Drink 4 oz. of this juice right after a meal.

Activated Charcoal

You can also use **activated charcoal**, to check your transit time. Here's how,

- Take 6 - 12 capsules (1.5 - 3 grams of charcoal)
- Take with 8 ounces of water

- Take these capsules between meals or right after a bowel movement
- Use Requa, activated charcoal

Checking Your Stools

When you have your next bowel movement, check your stools. When you drink chlorophyll, your stools will be green. With beets, your stools will be red. With Activated charcoal, they will be black. With corn, you will see undigested corn.

The time it takes for your stools to show color is your transit time. Again, you are looking for a transit time of 16 to 22 hours. If this time is less, your time is short, and you may not be getting the nutrients you need, from your food. If your time is long, your may have constipation and Candida.

Measure your transit at least two times before you start your acne program.

In the chapter for eliminating constipation, you will find ways to correct your transit time.

Chapter Summary

Here are the main points from this chapter.

You need to **check your transit time**. This is the time it takes your food to travel through your digestion system, from mouth to anus.

You can use **chlorophyll, beets, corn, or charcoal** to do this test. Prepare a chlorophyll-lemon or beet juice drink and take it right after a meal. Then, look at your next bowel movement and check for green or red stools. When green or red stools show up, determine your transit time. With charcoal, your stools will be black.

A good transit time can range from 16 to 22 hours. If this time is greater than 24 hours, you can consider yourself slightly constipated. The longer your transit time is the more severe your constipation.

Chapter 9: Testing For Thyroid Function

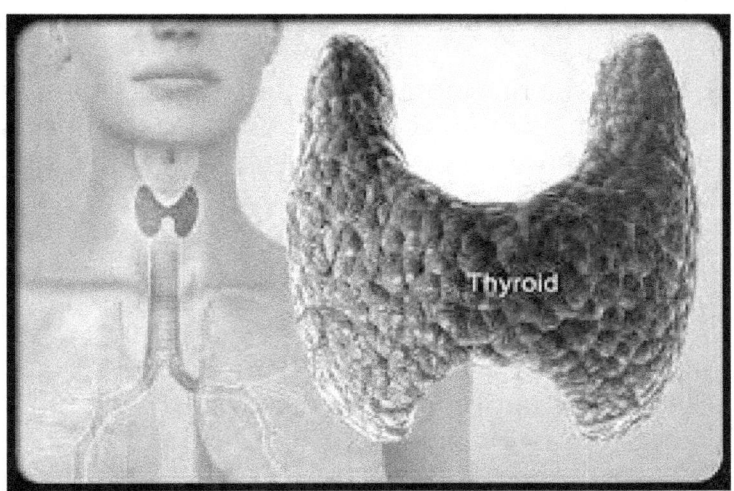

Thyroid Test

Here is a thyroid test you can do in your home. It's called the Barnes Basal Temperature Test. This test is not to be considered an absolute accurate test for determining whether you have a thyroid condition. It is a test that can suggest whether you need to go see a doctor for further thyroid tests. It is a test, to see if the symptoms you have correspond to hypo or hyper thyroidism.

Here's how to do the Test

It is best to use a mercury thermometer. Unfortunately, these thermometers are now banned. So, you need to use a digital thermometer. If you do have a mercury one, then shake it down, so the mercury level is below 90 degrees F, just before you go to bed.

If you don't have a thermometer, go to a drug or medical supplies store and ask for a Basil Temperature Thermometer to measure body temperature, for a thyroid test.

Do this test, when you first wake up in the morning, without moving much. Grab your digital thermometer and turn it on.

Place the tip of the thermometer in the deepest crease in your underarm. Then, wait for it to beep. If it does not beep, keep it there for 5 minutes. If you are using a glass thermometer, leave it in your underarm for 10 minutes.

Record your temperature. Do this test for three days in a row and compute the average body temperature.

If you have a period, do not test during the first five days of your period. Wait until the sixth day to start. All others can test any time, during the month.

Here is how to interpret your results.

- 97.8 to 98.2 F (is considered normal thyroid function) or 36.5 to 36.8 °C

- 97.6 F (hypothyroidism) or 36.4°C and below

- 98.3F (indicates possible hyperthyroidism) or 36.8°C and below

Hypothyroidism is an under active thyroid. This means that your thyroid is not releasing enough thyroxin to metabolize or digest your food at the cellular level.

Hyperthyroidism is when you are producing too much thyroxin.

If you have been diagnosis with thyroid problems, it would be a good idea to do this basal temperature test, before you start taking drugs. This would serve as your base temperature. As you take drugs, continue to monitor your temperature, to see if you have any changes. This will help you determine if the drugs you are using are helpful.

Remember, this temperature test is not absolutely perfect, so take readings for three days or more and compute an average reading. This average will be a better gauge of the accuracy of this test.

What is Goitrongen?

Your thyroid needs iodine to work well. Without iodine, you will develop goiter, an enlargement of the thyroid. When this happens, your thyroid hormones decreased and you tire easily and lack energy.

There are foods that have been identified as "goitrogens," which prevent iodine from being used in the thyroid. These foods are:

- Sweet potato
- Cabbage
- Cauliflower
- Turnips
- Rutabaga
- Canola Oil
- Cassava
- Pine Nuts
- Mustard
- Millet
- Soybeans

- Peanuts

However, if you cook these foods, then the goitrogenic properties are disabled.

Thyroid Diet

Beta Carotene

First, your diet must be rich in beta carotene. Beta carotene, a carotenoid, is an antioxidant and is the yellow, orange, or red in plants, fruits, and vegetables. When you eat food that is rich in carotene, your body converts it to vitamin A.

So why not take vitamin A supplements? Yes, you can take vitamin A supplements, but you must not take an excess of it, since it is toxic. When you eat beta carotene food, your body only converts the amount of carotene to vitamin A that it needs.

Also, when you eat carotene foods, they are packed with vitamins, minerals, antioxidants, and other nutrients that are balanced, with the right amount of beta carotene that your body needs.

Beta Carotene powers up your immune system and protects your thyroid cells from free-radical damage. Studies have shown that beta carotene reduces your risk of developing cancer.

Use the following foods in your recipes for breakfast, lunch, dinner, or snacks. They can be in the form of fresh salads, puddings, juices, or smoothies.

Spices

Spices are high in beta carotene. Because they are dried, the carotene is more concentrated. Use these spices in your cooking. These spices are listed in the order of highest carotene concentration.

- Paprika

- Cayenne pepper

- Chili powders

- Marjoram

- Sage

- Coriander

- Parsley

- Oregano

- Cumin

- Curry powder

- Fresh basil

- Fresh thyme

Sweet potatoes, boiled

Sweet potatoes are one of the highest foods in beta carotene. These can be used as snacks or puddings, or smoothies.

It is best to boil sweet potatoes instead of baking them. Once boiled, you can mix them slightly with other milks, such as rice dream or almond milk. Then you can add a touch of honey and cinnamon.

Carrots

Carrots are the king of vegetables. You can juice them and combine them with many other green vegetable juices to make them more palatable. Carrots are the vegetable you should be eating daily. Eat them both slightly cooked and raw, but cooked gives you more nutrition than raw.

Red bell peppers

Use the different color bell peppers and other chili peppers in your soups to get a high level of beta carotene. You can also use bell peppers in your salad. Use Tabasco sauce on your breakfast eggs or on other dishes you like.

Tomato Powder

If you can find tomato powder, add it to your soups. You can also cut up tomatoes and add them to your soups. Use tomatoes and tomato sauce any way you like.

Greens

These are the greens to concentration on. You can use them in salad, soups, or juices. When you juice them, add 1/2 to 3/4 carrot juice. You can experiment, with the amount of carrot juice you use. You may want to add a bit of apple juice to sweeten the taste.

Dandelion leaves, Kale, Spinach, turnip greens, mustard greens, and collards.

Lettuces to use in your salads are the dark green and red lettuces. The more orange and red color they have the better. Other vegetables to eat are asparagus, broccoli, and Chinese cabbage.

Pumpkin and Squash

Most people know how to use pumpkin. Pumpkin and squash can also be used in soups.

Fruits

The fruits that have the highest beta carotene are,
- Dried apricots

- Raw apricots
- Dried peaches
- Raw red cherries
- Grapefruit
- Mango
- Plums
- Plantains
- Raw guavas

Drugs that Interfere with Beta Carotene

There are some drugs that interfere with your absorption of beta carotene. And sometimes beta carotene will interfere with the effectiveness of a drug.

Statins – if you are taking statins, beta carotene can interfere with the effectiveness of Zocor and niacin.

Cholesterol-lowering drugs – cholestyramine and colestipol, can decrease your blood levels of beta carotene by up to 40% Weight control supplements – Orlistat, Xenical, and Alli can decrease your absorption of beta carotene by up to 30%.

Vitamin C

The next thing you need to concentration on is getting more vitamin C into your body. Many of the foods high in beta carotene are also high in vitamin C, so this makes it easy to get more vitamin C, when you concentration on beta carotene foods.

Here are the foods high in vitamin C.

Combine the juice of these three fruits – orange, grapefruit, and lemon. Use a hand juicer to prepare a fresh citrus juice drink. Take one fruit of each and juice it. You can drink this first thing in the morning.

Chapter Summary

Here are the main points from this chapter.

Check your thyroid function. This test is a good test to do and is fairly reliable. It can tell you, if your thyroid is overactive or underactive.

You need a good functioning thyroid, since you want to make sure your cells are getting the nutrition they need, to function properly. Also your thyroid puts out thyroid hormones, and it's good to eliminate any hormonal imbalances, you might have.

This **thyroid test** is easy to do. All you need is a digital thermometer, which you use to measure your morning underarm temperature. After you do this for 3 to 4 days in a row, you can get an idea, if you have hypothyroidism, low thyroid function, or hyperthyroidism, high thyroid function.

Getting rid of body acids will help your thyroid function better. In the following chapters, you will see how to eliminate acid from your body.

Thyroid Diet

If your tests show a thyroid imbalance, use the recommended diet.

First, you have to start eating those foods that are high in beta carotene. Then, you want to supplement your diet with 4000 to 5000 mg of vitamin C.

Make sure that you are not using statins, cholesterol drugs, or weight loss supplement, since they can reduce the effectiveness of beta carotene.

Chapter 10: Do You Have Candida?

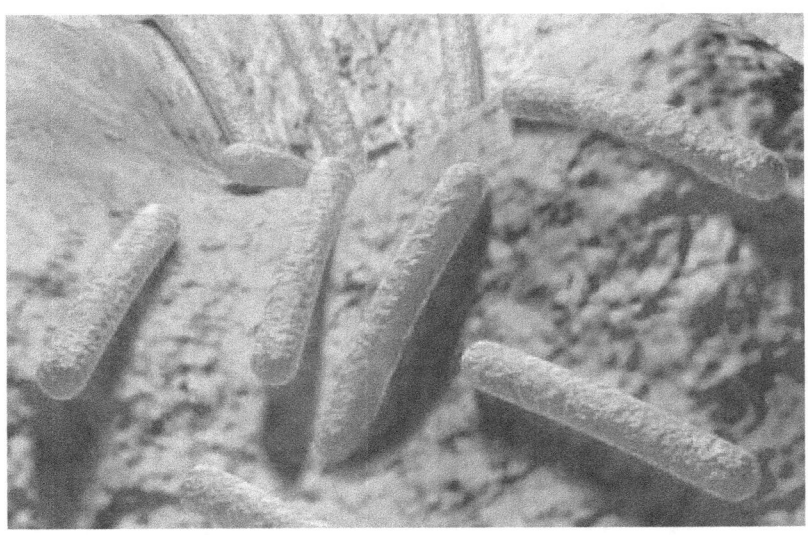

Candida Water Test

Candida is a micro-organism that is found in your colon, various body areas, and vagina. Candida always exists in your body. So, the only thing you can do is weaken it and in some cases eliminate it, so that your good bacteria can become dominant.

Here is a test that will indicate if you might have Candida. It's not an absolute diagnostic test, but it will give you an indication of the dominance of Candida in your body.
Start with a glass filled with reverse osmosis water. Then, first thing when you wake up, gather some saliva in your mouth and spit into the glass of water.

Here's what to look for, after waiting for 30 minutes.

If your saliva floats on top of the water chances are you don't have a severe case of candida. You may still have candida, but not as severe as the next tests suggestion.

If your saliva has stringers hanging or suspended cloudy specks, this indicates you have candida. If your saliva floats to the bottom of the glass, this test indicates you have severe candida.

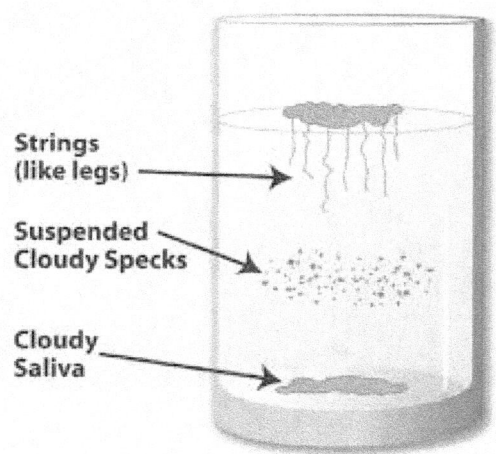

If you have candida, the only way to suppress it, is to change your diet, get more oxygen into your body, and drink herbal teas that kill it. But, drinking herbal teas that kill Candida, may not eradicate all the Candida.

Candida Sesame Seed Test

Here is another way to test for Parasites and Candida. In an 8 oz. of distilled water, add 2 tablespoons of whole sesame seeds. Drink this mixture without chewing the seeds.

This test is similar to the Transit Time Test. Keep track of the time it takes for these seeds to show up in your stools. If it takes more than 27 hours for these seeds to show up in your stools, than chances of you have Parasites and Candida are high.

When you are constipated and food remains too long in your colon, Parasites have a chance to lay their eggs and their eggs have time to hatch.

How to Tell If You Have Yeast or Parasites

There are many symptoms directly or indirectly associated with Candida and parasite overgrowth. If you have several of these symptoms, there is a really good chance that you have an infestation or overgrowth.

Symptoms of Candida and Parasite Overgrowth:

- Lowered immune system and constant illness
- Rectal itching, especially at night
- Frequent vaginal yeast or recurring bladder infections
- Sores on your mouth, lips or white spots inside the *mouth*
- Constant tiredness, difficulty sleeping, and waking up
- Toe fungus, athletes foot, Psoriasis, or eczema
- Bloating and gas, Constipation or diarrhea, Intestinal cramps
- Sensitivity to food, chemicals, cigarette smoke, or allergies
- Rashes or itching around genitals in men or women

- Food cravings, especially for sweet or carbohydrates
- A History of antibiotic use, steroids, contraceptive, high sugar

- Muscle or joint aches, floaters or spots before your eyes
- Brain fog or mental fuzziness, Anxiety or depression
- Menstrual irregularities, including heavy bleeding, cramps, PMS, or an ovulation
- Use of fluoride or consumption of fluoridated water

Candida Diet

Eat a diet that minimizes the strength of candida. In this diet, avoid,

- bread with yeast
- dairy products
- alcohol
- vinegar
- pickled food
- preserves; jams
- canned fruits and vegetables
- dried fruits, peanuts
- melons
- all foods that have sugar, artificial sweeteners, or flour
- cakes,
- biscuits, sweet drinks
- sugar
- honey, if you have a severe case

Here are some foods that you can eat for candida.

- If you have a mild case of candida, a slight amount of honey in your herbal tea is ok.
- You can eat two to three fruits per day, unless you have severe candida.
- Eating pure unprocessed oats is ok.
- You can eat un-sweeten yogurt for the probiotics.
- You can eat garlic, onions, leeks, and radishes. These have natural antibiotic properties.
- The best vegetables to eat are broccoli, cabbage, cauliflower.
- Use ginger in your cooking and tea.

The diet listed here is similar to other diets you will find in other chapters.

Best Candida Supplement

One of the best supplements to use to fight Candida is olive leaf, oregano, or wormwood, which you can find as a capsule or extract. Take the amount as indicated on the label.

Chapter Summary

Here are the main points from this chapter.

Do a saliva test, to determine if you have mild or severe candida. If you test positive for candida, the next chapter gives you ways to minimize your Candida level.
Use a glass of reverse osmosis water for the saliva test. Do the test 3 days in a row, so you can make sure of the results.

Also, do sesame seed test.

Use a **Candida diet** to minimize the strength of Candida in your body. Check out the list of foods not to eat and to eat, when you have Candida.

Chapter 11: Getting Rid Of Candida and Parasites

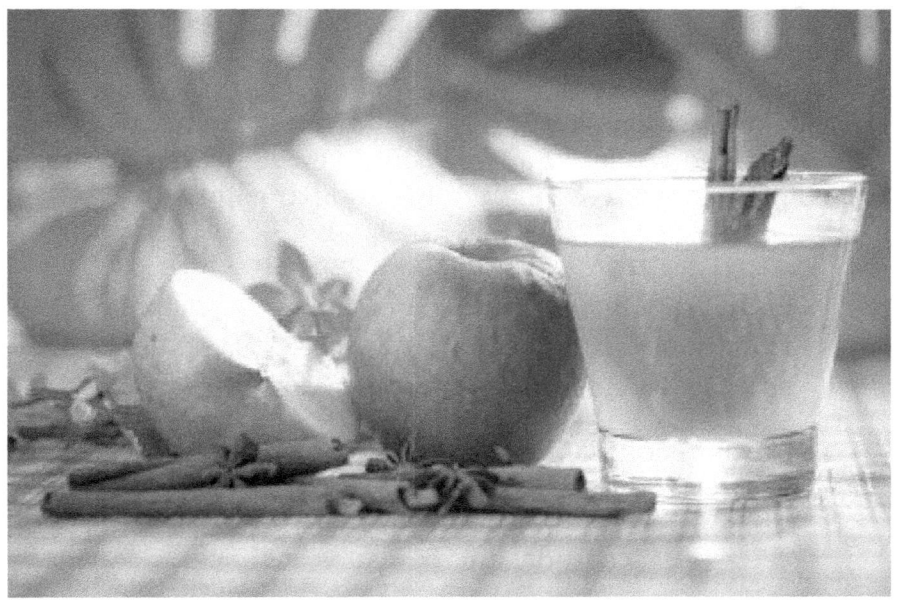

Alkaline Body Kills Pathogens

Making your body more alkaline will help you to eliminate parasites. It takes time to make your body alkaline, which requires eating specific fruits and vegetables. The transformation of changing your acid body into an alkaline body can take up to a year or
more. But, as you start changing your diet, your body will slowly start becoming less acidic.

Just assume you have parasites, since there are no tests that can detect all the parasites you might have. The best you can do is to reduce the quantity and the variety of parasites that you have.

The best way to get rid of parasites is to make your body uncomfortable for them to live in. To do this you need to have an alkaline body, bring in more oxygen into your blood, change your diet, stop eating sugar products, and drink specific herbal remedies.

Diet Changes

There are quite a few things you can do, to reduce an excess of Candida and parasites. Here is a list of things to do. Do these daily for three weeks. Each day that you use these methods, you will have a decrease in Candida and parasites.

1. Avoid eating sweets and sugars, fructose, starches, grains, and fruits, milk, and fat. This includes sugar from honey, fruits, candy, sweet breads, artificial sugar, sucrose, fructose, maple syrup, and so on.

2. Always cook vegetables and protein with garlic.

3. Include probiotics in your diet, since beneficial bacteria keep yeast, candida, and parasites in check.

4. Take Kyolic, an aged garlic supplement, after each meal.

5. Start using apple cider vinegar. Use 1 teaspoon in a small amount of water. Do this three times a day. If you eat a fresh salad, add a tablespoon of this cider to it.

6. Take a probiotics between meals, but do not take it within one hour of using apple cider vinegar. You can also eat unflavored yogurt or goat yogurt that has good bacteria.

Cinnamon Tea

Drink a tea of cinnamon. Add 1/2 teaspoon of cinnamon into

hot or cold water and drink it three times a day.

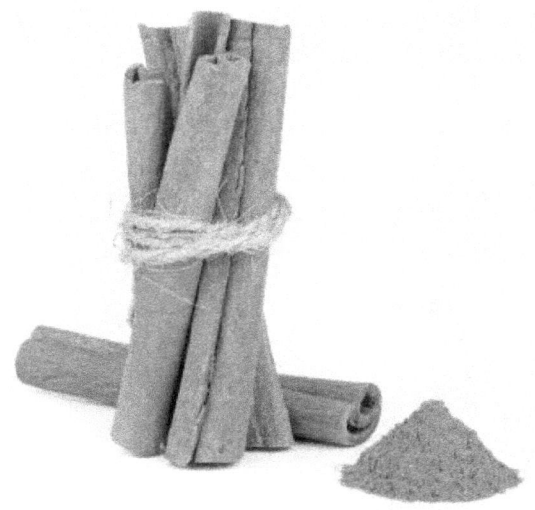

Vitamin

Use 5000 mg vitamin C every day, spread out in three doses. If you have diarrhea with this dose, just lower the dose, until your symptoms go away.

Diatomaceous Earth

Diatomaceous Earth has an amazing power, to kill parasites. Use 1 teaspoon per day in 8 ounces of water. You can work up to one tablespoon per day. Make sure you use a high quality food-grade Diatomaceous earth.

Coconut oil

Use coconut oil in your cooking. Use pure coconut oil for human consumption in your salads. You can add a tablespoon of this oil into your hot tea of choice.

Use olive and flax seed oil in your salads.

Herbal Remedies

Use a tea of the following herbs. You can mix two or three of these herbs together, to make a strong tea.

The herbal remedies that are effective in killing parasites are:

- Wormwood
- Black walnut
- **Oregano leaf or oil**
- Peppermint
- Rosemary
- **Olive leaf extract**
- Grape fruit seed extract

Here's how to make a tea or an infusion.

- Boil 2 to 3 cups of distilled water (more if you want)
- Turn off the heat
- Add one topping tablespoon of the herbs you mixed
- If using only one herb, add one topping tablespoon
- Mix the herb (s) into the water
- Let tea sit for 10 minutes (longer for a strong tea)
- Strain the tea

After the tea cools, drink 1/4 cup to 1/2 cup. Save the rest in a thermos to drink two more times during the day. Add a little bit of honey, if you like.

Pumpkin seeds were used by Native Americans to get rid of parasites. Use them for snacks frequently over a period of 3 weeks.

Sweating to Remove Parasite Toxins

As you eat and drink these various foods and teas to rid yourself of parasites, exercise to the point of sweating. This brings more oxygen into your blood and helps get rid of parasite.

If you take birth control pills, estrogen feeds your Candida bacteria. You have to decide what you want to do during the week you are trying to control your Candida bacteria.

Sugar and Candida

The main thing that creates an overgrowth of Candida in your body is sugar. The second is antibiotics. So, limit your use of sugar. If you have used antibiotics a lot, then it's time to take probiotics, to replace your good bacterium that was destroyed by the antibiotics you once took.

Chapter Summary

Here are the main points from this chapter.

Pathogens don't like an **alkaline body**. They prefer an acid body. When they find one, they multiple and dominate your good bacteria.

Because parasites feed on sugars, fruit sugars, fats, and oil, a new diet is outlined that will help you control and eliminate many of the parasites that you have.

For the **next three week,** keep this parasite diet to get rid of most of your parasites.

In this diet, the first thing to eliminate is eating sugar from honey, fruits, candy, sweet breads and so on.

Then, include **apple cider vinegar and cinnamon** in your

diet.

Look over the **herbs** that can help eliminate your parasites and create a tea to drink every day.

Chapter 12: Eliminating Your Constipation

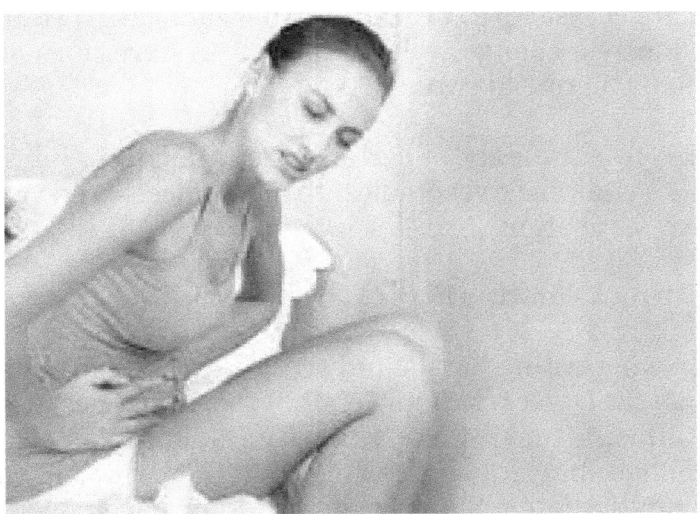

Start Eliminating Your Constipation

If you are constipated, you need to become regular; otherwise, it will be difficult to get rid of your acne. You should have from one to two bowel moments per day, and two is better.

The rule of thumb is, if you eat three meals each day, you should have three bowel movements each day. Typically, bowel movements come around 30 – 45 minutes after your meal.
What you eat at 8 am in the morning should promote a bowel movement the next day at 8 am. To eat food and eliminate the waste, should take around 16 to 22 hours.

Preventing constipation will require a change in the way you eat, exercise, and think – a lifestyle change - and this can sometimes be difficult, but it's something good. It requires a new mind-set and plenty of will power. Don't wait until you have an illness to change your mind-set. If you are ill, then this change is necessary now.

If you are using drugstore laxatives for constipation, then a change is necessary, to prevent further damage to your colon. With a lifestyle change, you can expect to have normal bowel movements, in one to two weeks.

You need to eat plenty of certain fiber, moisture, lubrication, minerals, vitamins, vegetables, fruits, juices, and water to prevent constipation.

Preventing Constipation

The following eating habits and lifestyles will help, to prevent constipation. Don't try to make all of these changes at once. It is too difficult. Make these changes gradually. Not only will these changes prevent constipation, but they will help you with your acne diet later. So, even if you don't have constipation, start changing over to this diet.

- Drink plenty of water
- Eat fewer processed carbohydrates
- Eat more nutritious food
- Eat plenty of fiber
- Eat the good oils
- Reduce emotional upsets– at home, office, and business
- Exercise regularly
- Feed the good bacteria
- Get plenty of rest and sleep
- Keep your colon acidic
- Take a good mineral supplement

- Use digestive enzymes

Drinking Plenty of Water

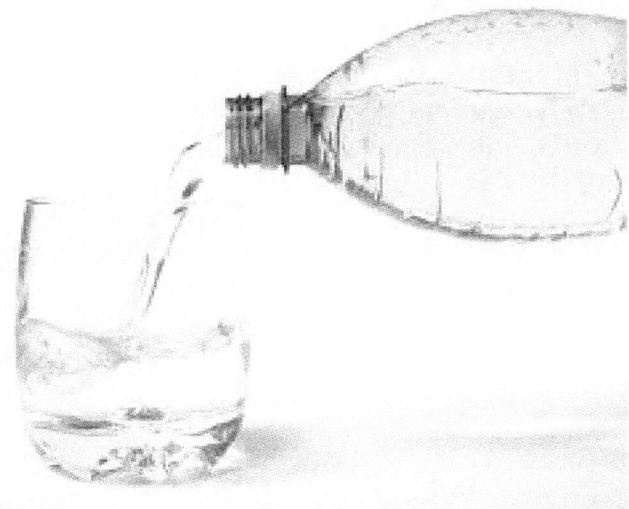

Drink plenty of water and it does not have to be eight glasses a day. But you need plenty of water to wash out body toxins as you detoxify. You have to sense when you are thirsty and drink water then.

Your body needs plenty of distilled water every day, to eliminate toxins from inside and outside its cells and from your blood. When you don't drink enough water, your body becomes dehydrated and will pull excess water out of your fecal matter, in your colon. This causes your fecal matter to become dry and more difficult to move through your colon.

Drinking Water with Meals

Drink water 30 minutes before meals, to help increase your stomach acid for the coming meal.

When you have your meals, don't drink water, since this water will dilute your stomach acid. This will reduce your ability to digest protein. During meals, drink only room temperature water, when food accumulates in your throat.

Drink a minimum of two quarts of water each day. You can add fresh squeezed lemon or small amounts of other juices to the water you drink, so that the water does not taste bland.

This way, you will be able to drink more water, at least two quarts each day. Or, you can make a ginger or green tea to drink in the morning and afternoon, flavored with a touch of honey.

What is Considered Water?

Liquids or juices that do not have added salt or sugar can be considered water. Water for your body also comes from:

- Fruit juices and fruits
- Herbal teas
- Vegetables, vegetable juices and broths
- Distilled water

Water **does not** come from:
- Sodas
- Sweeten fruit juices
- Coffee with sugar
- Tea with sugar
- Facet water
- Power drinks
- Milk

Eat fewer Processed Carbohydrates

The foods you must avoid to prevent constipation are processed foods or junk food. They are foods you find in fast-food restaurants and mini-marts. These foods have little fiber and are filled with chemical additives that cause your body to malfunction.

All dry foods such as bread, biscuits, bagels, crackers, bran, powdered foods, are difficult to move through your colon and can lead to constipation.

Processed foods cause constipation, since these foods lack fiber, nutrients, minerals, and enzymes. Consider all food products that come in bags, plastic, cans, and other containers processed foods. These foods contain excessive sugars, salt, coloring, dyes, hydrogenated oils, flavor enhancers, preservatives, MSG, and many other unknown chemicals.

Here are some of the foods to avoid:

- Alcohol, wine, and caffeine

- Processed foods

- Coffee

- Dairy products – eggs, milk, cheese butter

- Fried foods

- Excess meat

- Raisin Bran

- Refined sugar

- Regular tea – is rich in tannins, which helps diarrhea, but acts to hold back bowel movements.

- Salt

- Sodas

- Starch
- Sweets
- Cooked eggs, pasteurized milk, overcooked meat
- Mashed potatoes with gravy
- Overcooked carbohydrates
- Lipton or black Tea

Coffee

Coffee and tea have a tightening affect – astringent – on your colon, and this produces constipation. Drinking coffee on some occasions can have the opposite effect and promote a bowel movement.

Coffee or tea is not a recommended drink, when you have constipation or when you are trying to prevent constipation. This is not true for most herbal teas, which do not contain caffeine.

Caffeine can be found in,

Ground percolated coffee, 8 oz --------200 mg

Brewed tea, 8 oz ----------------------- 75 mg

Soft drinks ------------------------------ 40 mg

Chocolate ------------------------------- 10 – 40 mg

Painkillers ------------------------------ 60 mg

Fried Foods

Eating meat, bacon, sausage, and other fatty foods are constipating. These foods and others like butter, cheese, and eggs provide an excess of saturated fat and cholesterol that can easily stick to your colon walls. Cholesterol clings to your colon walls, just as it does in your arteries and organs.

Meat

All kinds of meat contain no fiber, and this makes them constipating. Meat moves slower through your colon than other foods. Since people eat a lot of meat at one sitting, undigested proteins usually make their way into your colon, which is fermented by bad bacteria. This decay creates a condition favorable for bad bacteria to multiple and is the start of many diseases that occur in your colon.

It is always best to eat plenty of uncooked vegetables when eating meat, carbohydrates or other food that contains no fiber. This provides fiber to help that food to move quickly through your colon.

Milk and Other Dairy Products

Dairy products are associated with constipation. This includes milk, cream soups, cheese, yogurt, some desserts, and baked goods. The best dairy product to eat is cottage cheese. It is the least harmful to your body of all the dairy products.

Eggs

Eggs, cheese, and butter are constipating and form toxic wastes, which poison your body. These foods can be eaten, but minimize their use.

Sodas

Soft drinks are high in phosphates. This chemical is used to dissolve sugar and to make soda taste better. When you drink soda, the phosphates combine with calcium. If you do not have enough calcium in your blood or lymph liquid, phosphates pull it out of your bones.

Drinking sodas leads to lower levels of calcium in your body. You need calcium to help keep your colon clean. Calcium is a major mineral that your body uses to keep your body alkaline.

Sweets

Most sweets are made from highly processed ingredients and an abundance of sugar. Because sweets are an unnatural food and contain no fiber, they contribute directly to constipation and should be avoided.

Sugar in sweets and in all other types of food has a deteriorating effect on your body. Sugar, in your body, can break down into many chemicals, one, which is alcohol. If you drink soda, the sugar in the soda supplies your body and brain with the alcohol ethanol.

Foods to Eliminate Constipation

Here is a list of food to eat when you have constipation. Rotate the foods and don't always eat the same food week after week.

Fruits

When you are trying to eliminate constipation, fruits are extremely effective. But as you get into the acne cleansing program, you will want to pick specific acid binding and cleansing fruits.

- Apricots, apples, cantaloupe, avocado
- Figs, blackberries, kiwi, strawberries
- Grapes, cherries, dates, peaches
- Raspberries, pears, pineapples, oranges
- Nectarines, coconuts, mangos, papayas
- Persimmons, plums, prunes, raisins

- Cranberries, elderberries, currants, gooseberries
- bananas

Vegetables

Vegetable are extremely helpful in eliminating constipation. Eating them raw, when possible, is the best way to get rid of constipation. Drinking their juice is also another way to use vegetables for constipation.

- collard greens, kale, dark green lettuce
- mustard greens, spinach, chard, cabbage
- dandelion greens, endives, corn, Brussels sprouts
- eggplants, asparagus, Jerusalem artichoke,
- rhubarb, rutabagas, carrots, celery, cauliflower
- peas, tomatoes, turnips, zucchini, beets
- potatoes, broccoli, pumpkin, squash
- bean sprouts, green beans, parsnip, sweet potatoes
- radish, peppers, onions, olives
- dulse, chicory, dandelion, parsley, watercress

Minimize cooking of vegetable, since it reduces or breaks down their fiber. Eat vegetables with skins, when possible.

Nuts, Beans, Grains

Nuts and seeds have many of the nutrients you need for good health. The contain plenty of fiber and omegas. Here is a list of the best nuts and seeds to eat.

- sesame seeds, walnuts, pumpkin seeds, pecans
- peanuts, black walnuts, almond, flaxseed

- lentils, broad beans, black beans
- pinto beans, kidney beans, chickpeas, lima beans, baked beans, navy beans
- millet, oats, barley, whole grains, spinach pasta
- whole wheat pasta

Beans Stop Constipation

Eat beans, since they are high in soluble and insoluble fiber. Eating them helps to prevent constipation and contributes to lowering your cholesterol. Beans become viscous, a thick heavy fluid, as they pass through your intestines. This viscous fiber fluid benefits your colon, sine it activates peristaltic action and promotes bowel movements.

Most all types of beans have close to the same nutritional value. So eat the type you enjoy and gain their benefit.

One cup of cooked pinto or kidney beans has around 20 grams of fiber per cooked cup. Lima and White beans have around 16 grams of fiber.

If you eat beans, avoid using canned beans. Here's how to cook in a crook pot.

- Rinse beans to remove dirt, tiny rocks, and bad beans
- Soak beans for 4-6 hours in water
- Dump the water from the soaked beans.
- Rinse beans again, using distilled or reverse osmosis water
- Place beans into the crook pot and cover with distilled water or reverse osmosis water

- Add a couple of garlic cloves and one cut up onion
- Add 2 to 3 capfuls of Eagle Brands Chili Powder or other chili powder that you like.

Turn crock-pot to low (not high) and cook beans for 8 hours or until beans are soft.

You can turn the crock-pot on low when you go to bed and in the morning you'll have cooked beans to eat for that day. Just make sure you have plenty of water covering your beans.

Eat Good Oils

Good oils such as olive, flaxseed, evening primrose, black currant, and borage seed provide lubrication to the lining of your intestines and colon. This lubrication of your colon and fecal matter is necessary for you to have regular bowel movements. Use these oils in place of mineral or castor oil.

Evening Primrose Oil - take 500 mg three times daily.

Omega-3 and Omega-6 are found in flax seeds and in fish, such as Alaskan salmon, tilapia, rainbow trout, cod and halibut.

Fish

Do not eat fish for dinner. It is ok for lunch. Fish is hard to digest, and you want to avoid foods that take too much time to digest, during the evening.

Fish Oil

Fish oil contains omega-3 fatty acids, which are essential for good health. It has these fatty acids in the form of EPA, Eicosapentaenoic acid and DHA, docosahexaenoic acid.

Fatty acids help reduce inflammation through prostaglandin production. Prostaglandins help reduce inflammation in your colon, which help make your colon work better and reduce the possibility of constipation.

Make sure when taking fish oil that is it is not fish liver oil. They are a different food product. Fish liver oil can elevate blood sugar and cholesterol levels, in some diabetics.

Note: Fish oil can increase the rate of bleeding, if you are using anticoagulant drugs such as warfarin, Coumadin, or platelet inhibiting drugs - aspirin or ticlopidine.

Recommend dose of fish oil is 1500 to 2000 mg each day.

Flax Seeds

Flax seeds fall in the top 10 healthy foods to live on. It contains a high-level of the omega-3 fatty acids that are essential for life. You cannot live without omega-3 fatty acids. Your diet must consist of a 3:1 or 4:1 ratio of omega-6 to omega-3. You must have 3 or 4 parts of omega-6 to 1 part of omega-3 in your diet.

So here is what you can do to get more omega-3 in your diet. Use 1-3 tablespoon of flax seed daily. Always grind these seeds with a coffee grinder. Then add them to your food.

- Add 1 to 2 teaspoon(s) to your smoothie
- Add 1 to 2 teaspoon(s) to your salad dressing
- Add 1 to 2 teaspoon(s) to your cereal

Use flax seeds without heating them. This preserves the nutritive value of this food and prevents its oxidation.

Garlic

Include raw garlic in your diet and in cooking. Garlic destroys harmful bacteria in your colon and penetrates your colon walls to loosen up accumulated waste.

Also, you can use aged garlic extract, which comes in a capsule. Aged garlic promotes the growth of good bacteria in your colon.

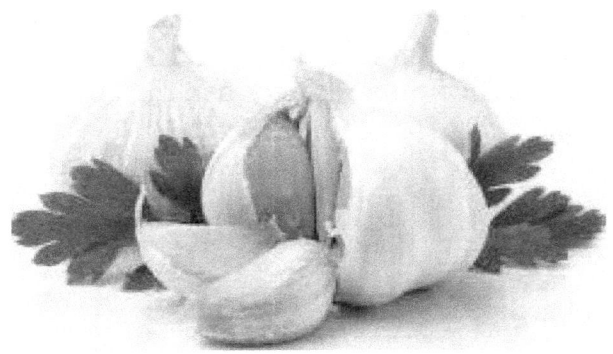

Exercise

Exercise is necessary for reducing or minimizing constipation. Here is what exercising does for your colon and body,

- Tones and strengthen your colon muscles
- Eliminates blood toxins by sweating.
- Stimulates your cells to eliminate waste, which is moved into your lymphatic system
- Reduces tension and anxiety
- Stimulates your colon wall cell structure to increase its metabolic rate and thus improve its function.

Daily walks, after a meal, stimulate your colon for bowel movements. In addition, walking strengthens and tones your colon walls. This prevents your colon from becoming misshaped when you, on occasion, become constipated.

There are many good exercises that stimulate and strengthen your body. Any type of exercise will be of benefit for your health. When your colon is toxic, exercises activate the lymphatic system to remove that toxicity.

Feed the Good Bacteria

The good bacteria, in your colon, are known by many names – good bacteria, micro flora, and probiotics. This bacterium is necessary for good colon and body health. The main bacteria in your colon are:

- Lactobacillus acidophilus
- Bifidobacterium bifidum
- Lactobacillus salivarius
- Bifidobacterium infantis
- Streptococcus faecium

Buy a probiotics that has only one or two of the main bacteria listed above. In some products, you will find Fructo-oligosaccharides, FOS, which helps to feed the good bacteria and promote their survival.

Cultured yogurt is a good way to get additional good bacteria into your colon. The best way to eat it is in-between meals. The best yogurt to eat is goat milk yogurt. It costs a bit more, but it is worth the health benefits you get from it.

Look for yogurt that says the bacteria culture was added after pasteurization. If the yogurt was pasteurized after the bacteria, culture was added, the good bacteria would have been destroyed.

Eat yogurt at least three times a week. You can add flax seed oil, berries, raisins, flax seed grounds, or other toppings that promote bowel movements.

The best way to get probiotics or good bacteria into your colon is to take a supplement, liquid or pill, between meals with distilled water. When probiotics are taken with food, food increases your stomach acid, which destroys the probiotic supplement.

Eating cultured vegetables is another way to get probiotics or good bacteria. Some flora-enhanced foods are:

- Sauerkraut
- Yogurt
- Kefir
- Miso
- Micro alga

Chapter Summary

Here are the main points from this chapter.

If your **transit time** indicted you have constipation, then follow the diet in this chapter for two to three weeks. This will help normalize your bowel movements. You want to have at least two bowel movements per day. But, make sure you don't use drugstore laxative for this cleanse. If you can get one bowel movement a day, this is a good start.

If your tests show that you are not constipated, you still need to start changing your diet as outlined in this chapter. Many of the diet concepts here will be used in diets outlined in other chapters.

Follow the list on how to **prevent constipation**. Start with drinking plenty of water and increase your intake of fiber. Use digestive enzymes and exercise.

Reduce your intake of carbohydrates and meat. Load up on vegetables and use fruits for snacks.

You have a **list of foods to avoid**. Follow this list consistently.

The idea here is to **eat more nutritious food and less junk food**. This chapter is packed with the right type of food to eat. Using this diet will not only help your constipation, but will set the stage for cleansing your body.

Don't try to apply all the dietary recommendations listed in this chapter in one week. Start by making one or two changes per day. Within 3 to 4 weeks, you will not have constipation.

Chapter 13: Cleansing To Stop Acne

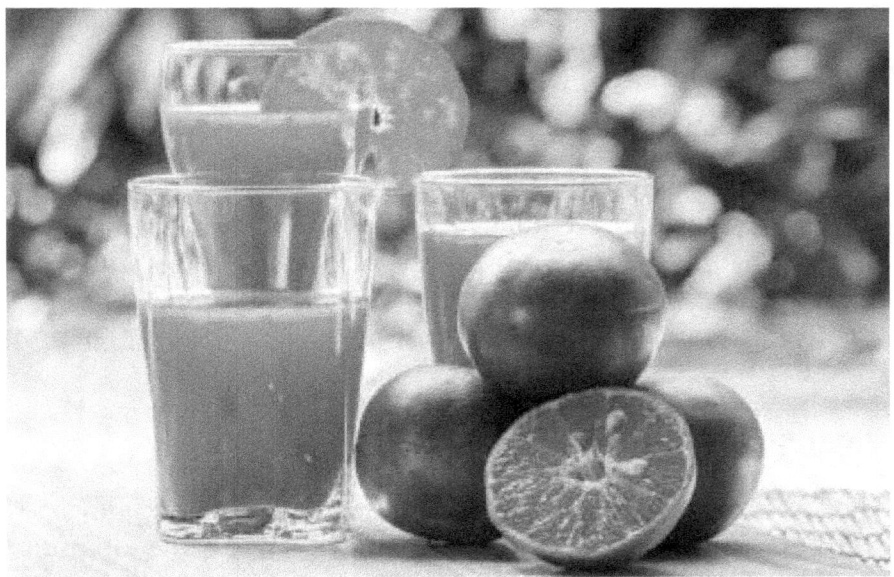

Cleansing Your Body

Cleansing your body of toxins is critical for your acne program. The cleaner your body is the fewer toxins will be pushed into your follicles and out of your skin. Your immune system will get stronger and will be able to deal with controlling parasite, toxins, and diseases.

If you are still slightly constipated, this cleanse will push out accumulated fecal matter in your colon, giving you a new start for having regular bowel movements.

Body Odor

If you have strong underarm or body odor, bad breath, and

stools that smell, you have a lot of toxins to get rid. All of these odors should not be strong. You will have them, but not to the point where you annoy people around you.

In her extensive book, Cooking For Healthy Healing, 1991, Linda Rector-page, N.D., Ph.D., talks about what a cleanse does,

"Fasting works by self-digestion. During a cleanse, the body in its infinite wisdom, will decompose and burn only the substances and tissue that are damaged, diseased, or unneeded, such as abscesses, tumors, excess fat deposits, and congestive wastes. Even a relatively short cleanse can accelerate elimination from the liver, kidneys, lungs and skin, often causing dramatic changes as masses of accumulated waste is expelled. Live foods and juices can literally pick up dead matter from the body and carry it away."

Cleanse Your Colon

The minimum time for this cleanse is three to four days. If you can do it long, five or seven days, you will gain more cleansing benefits. Doing this cleanse is not a cure all. During your program, you should this cleanse every month until your acne is gone.

As you start this cleanse, keep in mind that you don't have to do exactly what I have outlined here. Each person is different as to what they eat and what works for them, so chose the juices you like and setup the timeline that fits your life.

As you start this cleansing diet, you can develop symptoms that are uncomfortable. This may be a headache, running nose, gas, upset stomach, or a feeling of "not feeling good." This is caused by toxins being stirred up throughout your body and your body looking for a way to get rid of them.

After a few days, these unpleasant symptoms will go away. If they don't, and they get worse, then back off by one-half of everything you are doing. Temporarily, you might want to eat a small amount of protein or carbohydrates to settle your stomach. Then, you can start your cleanse again.

With this cleanse, you may see more acne breakouts. But, this will stop and you will see fewer breakouts, as you continue with your cleanse.

Things to Do Daily

Take a good supplement of calcium, magnesium and vitamin D3. The magnesium and vitamin D3 will help you absorb more calcium. You need more calcium during cleansing, so that it can help you neutralize toxic acidic waste.

Start this cleanse on a Saturday, Sunday or any other day that you don't have to go anywhere. You will be going to the bathroom all day, and at times you need to be there quick. After the first day or second your will get a feel for how often your need to reach a bathroom.

What to Buy For Your Cleanse

- Organic apple juice – 2 gallons
- Organic apples – 10 to 15 for three days
- Organic prune juice – one quart
- Supplement – Calcium-magnesium-D3

Day before the fast

The day before the fast, eat a large salad and two apples. This will give you plenty of fiber to scrub your colon walls, when you have a bowel movement the following day.

Night Before the Cleanse

If you are doing an Oxypowder cleanse, then around 6-8 pm, the day before you start your cleanse, take 4-5 Oxypowder capsules. Oxypowder takes about 12 hours to activate your colon, so you will not have a bowel movement at night.

In the next chapter, you will start your Body Cleanse.

Chapter Summary

In this chapter, you got the information on what you need to start your cleanse, in the next chapter.

This **cleanse will remove acids**, parasite excretions, and toxic matter from your blood, lymph, organs and tissue. This is a powerful cleanse, and you will notice your energy difference when you complete it.

Take a supplement of calcium-magnesium-D3 to help you neutralize body acids.

You now have a list of the juices, fruits, and supplements you need to buy for this cleanse. Make sure you use vitamin D3 and magnesium during this cleanse.

If you are going to use **Oxypowder** for your cleanse, take four to five capsule the night before your cleanse.

Chapter 14: Oxypowder Body Cleanse

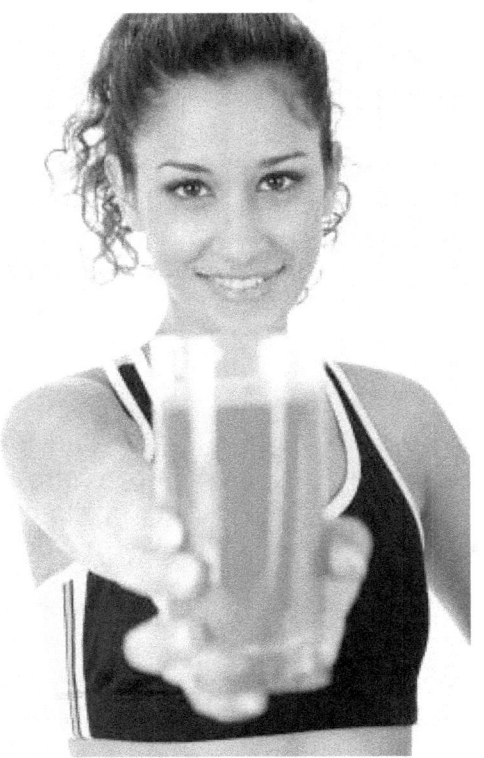

Two Different Body Cleanses

There are two different cleansing methods here. The first one is where you use **Oxypowder,** and the second one is where you use **Prune Juice**.   So, if you can't afford to buy Oxypowder, then you can use the prune juice cleanse. Both cleanses are effective.

Purpose of This body cleansing step is to:

- Remove toxins from your body
- Remove excess acids from your body

- Cleanse your colon
- Get rid of constipation
- Cleanse your lymph liquid of toxins
- Pull toxins out of your cells
- Purify your blood
- Give liver a rest so it can rejuvenate
- Improve your immune system

You should have all the material for your body cleanse, so let's get started.

Day before the Fast

The day before the fast, eat a large salad and two apples at dinner time. Eat very little protein or carbohydrates with this meal. This meal will give you plenty of fiber to scrub the walls of your colon, when you have a bowel movement the following morning.

Oxypowder Cleanse

If you have decided to use Oxypowder, take five to six Oxypowder pills, just before you go to bed. This will activate your first bowel movement, in the morning. Taking Oxypowder before bedtime will not wake you at night to go to the bathroom.

Oxypowder is not addictive nor a laxative, even though your bowel movements will be watery. Oxypowder uses oxygen to dissolve the fecal matter in your colon.

First Day of Cleanse: Morning

1. When you first wake up, take three to four capsules of Oxypowder.

2. Take only two Oxypowder capsules, if you want less bowel movement activity during the day.

3. Then, drink a chlorophyll drink of 1-2 oz of chlorophyll, the juice from one lemon, and the rest distilled or reverse osmosis water.

4. Prepare 16 oz or more of apple juice in a thermos, if you are going to work.

5. Add ½ to one teaspoon of powdered vitamin C to the thermos. You can use the powder in a vitamin C capsule.

6. Eat several pieces of watermelon or melons of any kind.

The chlorophyll drink will help neutralize toxins that are in body and colon. This will help to minimize toxic sickness feelings, as you cleanse. The lemon will help detoxify your liver.

The watermelon puts distilled water into your body. It is a diuretic, which pulls water out of your body and helps to cleanse your kidney. Also, the watermelon provides fiber to your colon, so that it can help the Oxypowder remove accumulated waste that attaches to your colon walls.

The vitamin C powder you put into your juice acts as a preservative and prevent the juice from becoming rancid, during the day.

Break Time

An hour or so after eating watermelon or other fruit, drink a glass of the juice you have prepared. Then, drink a glass of this juice every hour during the day.

Lunch

Eat a bowl of fresh fruits and drink a pure juice of any kind.

Dinner

Eat pieces of watermelon, cantaloupe, or other fruit. Continue drinking your prepared juice. You can also prepare any type of vegetable juice that you like.

Eat one small cantaloupe. Finish off your prepared juice drink, if you have not finished it by 5 pm, just dump the remaining prepared juice. If you have finished, then drink a juice of another kind. Do not drink anything at least one hour before your bedtime.

Take four to six capsules of Oxypowder, just before you go to bed.

Day Two of the Cleanse

Do the same thing you did on the first day.

If on the first day, you are having too many bowel movements, and it's interfering with your work, you can back off on the morning or night Oxypowder capsules. You can experiment with how many Oxypowder capsules are right for you and your work schedule.

Third Day of Cleanse

Do the same thing you did on the first day. But, now you should eat other fruits and vegetable in the morning and throughout the day. Also start a vegetable drink such as carrot and apple juice.

Fourth Day of Cleanse

On the fourth day, you will need to start your day early, so that you have time to activate a bowel movement, doing the following. You need to do this cleanse, when you don't work or on a Saturday. You can plan your cleanse to start on Wednesday so that this fourth day of cleansing is on Saturday.

- When you first wake up, here's what you do.

- Drink 2 to 3 cups, 8oz of prune juice

- Half an hour later drink 8 oz of apple juice

- A half-hour later, drink another 8 oz of apple juice.

- Every hour during the day, drink 8 oz of apple juice or any other juice.

After drinking the prune juice and apple juice, you will get an urgent call for a bowel movement. Be close to a bathroom at this time.

If you go to work, be ready to go to the bathroom frequently. If you cannot frequent the bathroom at work, you should start this cleanse, so that your prune juice day falls on Saturday or Sunday. .

The prune juice day is a powerful tool to purge out loose matter in your small intestine and in your colon. It activates your colon to produce strong peristaltic action to help clean out your colon. The prune and apple juice provides you with plenty of minerals and some vitamins to help neutralize acids in your body.

If you want to continue your cleanse for more days, here's what to do.

Fifth Day of Cleanse

When you first wake up, take three capsules of Oxypowder.

Do not drink the prune juice. Drink a chlorophyll drink or if you like you can add chlorophyll to a carrot-apple, or orange juice. Eat a bowl of fruit.

Repeat the fourth day of juices, fruits, and vegetables, except don't do the prune juice.

- Drink the following juices at these times:
- Orange juice 1 quart: as soon as you wake up
- Grape juice 1 quart near noon time
- Pineapple juice mid after noon
- Carrot-apple around 6 pm

Drink these juices slowly over an hour or so. Drinking this much juice at one time helps flush out your colon and provides with the minerals you need.

Sixth Day of Cleanse

Repeat the third day.

Eat fruits or vegetable juice for breakfast and lunch, and drink the juices you like during the day. Do not mix drinking fruit and vegetable juices.

Eat a green salad at the end of the day with some apple cider vinegar and olive oil.

Prepare a green salad with a variety of different fresh vegetables. You can add a small amount of flax seed oil, olive oil, and apple cider vinegar, as salad dressing. At the end of the day, take three capsules of Oxypowder.

Seventh Day of Cleanse

First thing in the morning drink a green drink – chlorophyll and the juice from one lemon.

Then, take three capsules of Oxypowder.

Eat plenty of raw green and other vegetables, with olive oil, flaxseed oil, and apple cider vinegar.

And drink fruit and vegetable juices throughout the day

At the end of the day take another three Oxypowder capsules.

When you finish your cleanse, you will want to start one month of probiotics, so that you can replace the good bacterium that was killed or that was flushed out during your cleanse.

Final Cleansing Suggestions

There you have it; a seven-day fruit and vegetable juice cleanse. You can do a three or four day cleanse, if you can't do a seven day cleanse.

If you do the 4 day cleanse on the fifth day, eat fruits, salad, and a little protein or carbohydrates.

Chapter Summary

Here's the chapter summary of the main points.

In this chapter, you learned how to do an **Oxypowder body cleanse.** Using Oxypowder, gives this cleanse added power, since the Oxypowder provides oxygen to your colon. This oxygen dissolves hard fecal matter in your colon. It will also kill all good and bad parasites and bacteria.

This cleanse is critical, since it will remove toxins from all parts of your body. It gives your liver a rest, so that it can rejuvenate itself.

Take four to six **Oxypowder Capsules the night before**

your cleanse. In the morning, you will have a watery bowel movement. Oxypowder is not a laxative or habit forming. Use it all month, after your cleanse, at one or two capsules per day.

The **first day of your cleanse** you will take more Oxypowder. And you will take your first chlorophyll drink. Then, you will eat some watermelon for breakfast. During the day, you will drink only apple juice, every hour on the hour.

During a break, you can eat watermelon or any other fruit or fruit juice. Do this for the first three days. You can also drink vegetable juices that you juice.

On the **fourth day,** you will use prune juice, in morning to clean out your colon with the minerals and nutrients.

You can continue to do this **cleanse for seven days,** if you are able. The longer you do this cleanse past three days the more benefit you will get.

Chapter 15: Prune Juice Body Cleanse

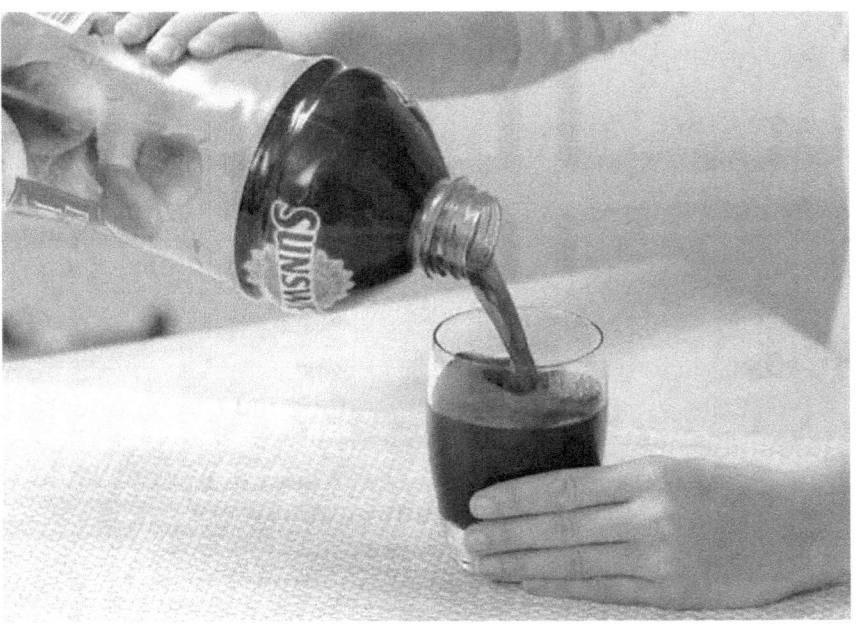

Second Way to Do a Body Cleanse

For this cleanse, you will need the following:

- Organic apple juice – one gallon
- Organic apples – 3 for one day, 12 apples for three days
- Organic prune juice – 1/2 gallon
- Organic Cherry juice – 1/2 gallon
- Carrots for your juicer or carrot juice – one quart or more
- Lemons, grapefruits, and oranges

The day before your body cleanse, eat a large salad and two apples for dinner. This will give you plenty of fiber, to scrub the walls of your colon, when you have a bowel movement the following day.

First Day of Colon Cleanse

Lemon Juice Drink

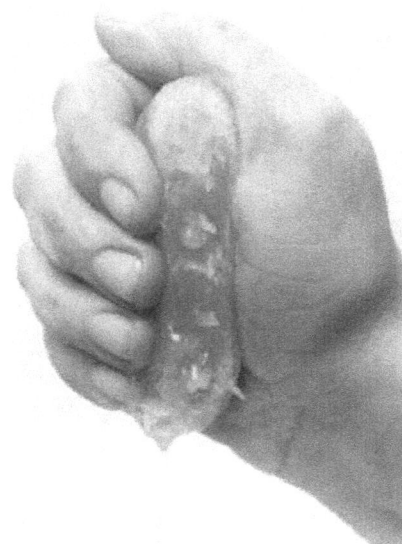

Every morning, when you first get up, drink a glass of slightly warm water with juice from one lemon.

This will remove mucus from your intestinal tract and detoxify your liver.
You can add some lime juice or grapefruit juice, if you like.

Prune Juice Colon Cleanse

- About 1/2 hour after your lemon drink, take three glasses of prune juice. Sip them slowly over 10 minutes.

- Now, wait 20 minutes, then drink 8 oz. of apple juice

- Wait another 30 minutes, and then drink another 8 oz. of apple juice.

- If you haven't sped to the bathroom yet, you will in a little while.

- After an hour, drink another 8 oz. of apple juice.

- Now every hour, during the day, drink a glass of apple juice, until the end of the day.

- You can eat a couple of apples during the day.

You can stop drinking apple juice around 5 pm. Now, you can drink different fruit or vegetable juices in place of apple juice. During the day, you can eat one or two apples in the morning and in the evening.

Second Day of the Colon Cleanse

During the second day, you can drink different kinds of juices and eat 2-6 apples. You can drink any kind of juice be it fruit or vegetable. A combination of apple and vegetable juices is good.

You can to eat watermelon, melon, oranges, grapefruit, and strawberries during the morning or day.

Drink your juice every hour or every 1 1/2 hours

Third Day of the Colon Cleanse

The third day is like the second day, where you can drink different kinds of juices and eat 2-6 apples or other fruit.

On this day, you can eat other fruits, like mango, watermelon, cantaloupe, and pineapple. At the end of this day, you can eat a salad with a variety of vegetables.

Fourth Day of Colon Cleanse

In the morning, start with your lemon drink and your fruit breakfast. For lunch prepare a vegetable soup without meat. For Dinner, prepare a large salad with apple cider vinegar, flax seed oil, and olive oil dressing.

Fifth Day, after the Cleanse is Done

After you have finished your three or four day cleanse, start eating soft foods for a day or so. Here are some of the foods you can eat,

- Baked potato
- Fruit salad
- Fruit smoothie
- Light soup
- Oatmeal, multi-grain cereal
- Salad
- Natural Yogurt

You can prepare a fruit smoothie with four special nutrients as listed in the last chapter of this book.

Here is a list of juices and vegetables you can use for your cleanse.

Juices to Drink

Apple, Grape, Cherry, Orange, Lemons, Grapefruit, Pineapple, blueberry, blackberry, Cranberry, raspberry, combination of berries, Grapefruit, Carrot, Carrot-Apple, Carrot-Chlorophyll, Orange-Chlorophyll, Celery, Goat's milk, raw milk

Use a combination of different juices, to get the benefit of their nutritional value. There are some juices that are not as sweet as others, so use them also.

Vegetables to Eat

Dark-green lettuce, Beets, Carrots, Cucumbers, Cabbage, Tomatoes, Parsley, Onions, Spinach, Turnips, Asparagus, Garlic

Try to use those vegetables that you typically don't use. These vegetables will help you detoxify more. Stay away from the iceberg lettuce, since it has little nutritional value. You can use romaine and butter lettuce, but try to use some of the dark-green leafy ones.

Fruits to Eat

Watermelons, Cantaloupes, Casaba Melon, Strawberries, Cherries, Pears, Coconuts, Oranges, Peaches, Mangos, Apples, Bananas, Avocados

Chapter Summary

Here is another way to do your body cleanse, without Oxypowder. Do this **prune juice cleanse** for four days.

Buy the **list of juices**. You may want to buy other dark juices, like pomegranate or grape juice. These dark juices have more antioxidants.

The **night before your cleanse**, eat a big salad. The next morning start out with a warm lemon juice drink.

Start your prune juice cleanse as outlined in this chapter. Then, drinking juices on the hour all day. In the evening, you can eat apples or a fruit salad.

On the **third and fourth day** you can eat a salad, but during the day continue with the juices or fruits.

Chapter 16: Cleansing Your Kidneys

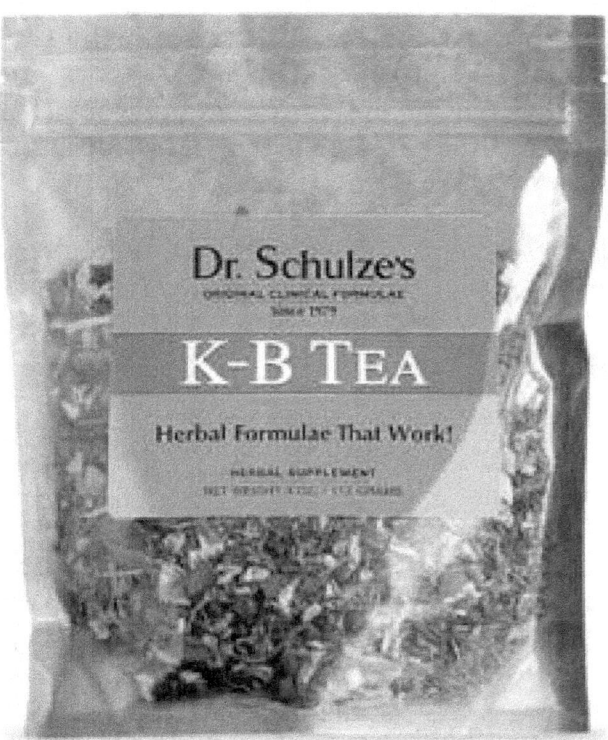

Kidney cleanse

To do an effective kidney cleanse, you need to have good functioning kidneys. This cleanse will remove toxic material out of your blood and flush and detoxify your kidneys. Your kidneys will take these toxins and route them out of your body as urine. If your kidneys are weak, this cleanse can't remove all the toxic material out of your blood or kidneys. The toxic material will stay in your blood and get routed back into your body where it can do damage.

So here are two ways to do kidney cleansing.

Dr. Schulze's Kidney Cleansing Kit
The easiest way to do a kidney cleanse is to buy Dr. Schulze's kidney-cleansing kit. Look for it on the Internet.

Buy the K-B Formula and the **K-B Tea**, which uses herbs that will help you flush and detoxify your kidneys and bladder. These herbs are diuretic and antiseptic for your entire urinary tract. In addition, they reduce urinary tract inflammation and dissolve kidney stones.

Some acne or certain skin conditions are really difficult to eliminate. Skin conditions are normally a result of weak, overworked, or toxic internal elimination organs.

Herbal Kidney Cleanse

If you can't afford Dr Schulze's teas, then this is an alternate way to cleanse your kidney.

Using herbs for kidney cleansing has been happening for hundreds of years. Here are some teas to make. Pick three of these herbs and make a tea. Drink one to three cups per day, during your kidney cleanse week.

1. Nettle tea – helps cleanse and support your kidneys and eliminate uric acid. The more acid you eliminate from your body the stronger your immune system becomes.

2. Green tea - has anti-inflammatory, astringent and diuretic properties.

3. Couch grass - Couch grass can partially dissolves kidney stones and has diuretic, demulcent and antibacterial properties.

4. Cornsilk - helps to flush out the kidneys and bladder

and ease inflammation.

5. Dandelion - works as a diuretic and cleanser by relieving fluid retention and detoxifying the kidneys

6. parsley - assists in keeping kidneys healthy and clean by eliminating waste and toxins.

Kidney Tonics

This is a tonic for your kidneys. Juice the following and drink one to two cups per day.

1. 1 cucumber
2. A handful of fresh parsley
3. 1 stalk of celery with leaves
4. Juice of one lemon
5. 1/2 inch piece of fresh ginger root

Beet Root Juice

This juice is a great body builder and helps to clean out your kidneys and gallbladder. The juice combination is: **beet, carrot, and cucumber juice**

Mix more carrot juice than beet or cucumber. Make different mixtures every day.

This juice can clear your blood of toxins and will help to rebuild your liver, kidney, lungs, heart, and brain.

Cranberry Concentrate

You can add drinking cranberry juice, for cleansing out your kidney. You can drink it regularly, during this program. It is best to buy a bottle of concentrate cranberry, thendilute it down to your taste, so that you can control the strength.

Kidney Detox Juice Drink

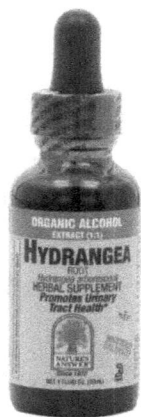

Here is an easy drink to make. Drink this every day, for a period of 3 weeks.

- 1 cup of apple juice

- 21 to 29 drops of **hydrangea root tincture**

Use organic apple juice, but what is best is fresh apple juice or juice that is not pasteurized.

Hydrangea is frequently used to treat malaria, enlarged prostate, kidney stones, blood sugar imbalances, and urinary tract infections in the bladder and kidneys.

Chapter Summary

Using **Dr. Schulze's kidney cleansing kit**, it the best way to cleanse your kidneys. It provides you with the right herbs to cleanse and support your kidney.

If you don't have Dr. Schulze's herbs, you can drink nettle tea, with two other herbs listed. All these herbs are diuretic and detoxifying.

You can also use the kidney tonic listed. This is a powerful drink to take.

Cranberry Juice can be used to cleanse out your kidney. This juice can be added to your juices to drink between meals.

You can also use **Hydrangea root** and apple juice to eliminate prostate or bladder or kidney infections.

Chapter 17: Cleansing your Liver

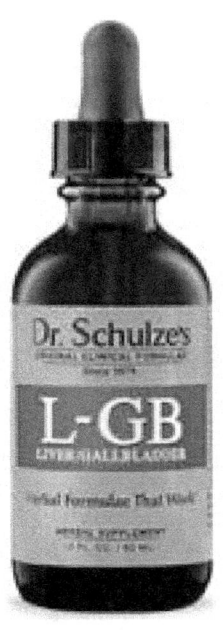

In this chapter, you will find the information to do a liver cleanse. In addition, you will find a diet that will help you support and cleanse your liver.

Information is provided on how important your liver is in clearing up your acne.

Dr. Schulze's Liver Gallbladder Cleanse

Using **Dr. Schulze's Liver cleanse** is the best way to do your liver cleanse.

About Your Liver

Your liver is central to how your body functions. If your liver is sluggish, clogged, or diseased, you will be open to many different diseases, such are constipation, high cholesterol, IBS, high blood sugar, asthma, skin rashes, acne, allergies and more.

If you have acne, your liver contributes considerably to this condition. For this reason, in this chapter, you will find out how you can get your liver back on track, so that it is not a factor in creating your acne.

Your liver is a detoxifying organ. Because of the tremendous pollution that is in the environment and in everything you eat and drink, your liver is usually overloaded. Your liver is called upon to eliminate all of this pollution and at some point becomes unable to do this. When this happens, your liver allows various pollutants to enter your blood. This is when your other organs become compromised, and cells and body liquids become contaminated. Over time, you become diseased.

Your liver uses the channels of elimination, to rid your body of incoming toxins. It uses the colon, kidney, lungs and skin to move toxins out of your body. When all of your elimination channels are overworked, your skin is bound to have its share of toxic overload.

Liver distress

So what causes your liver to become distressed? Your liver becomes distress, when you eat processed foods, food in packages, sugar, artificial sweeteners, caffeine, dips, breads, cookies, and hydrogenated oil. It becomes distressed when you don't have a healthy diet.

A Liver Diet

One of the best ways to keep good liver health is to limit the use of alcohol, sugar, and saturated fat.

Your liver likes fresh, whole fruits and vegetables or cooked lightly. It likes cooked grains and legumes, raw nuts, and seeds.

It likes food with fiber. You need around 35 grams of fiber every day. In your colon, fiber absorbs excess cholesterol and estrogen and prevents it from being reabsorbed into your blood. When reabsorbed estrogen gets into your blood, it becomes active and disturbs the balance of your hormones.

Fiber is also necessary to prevent constipation. Fiber absorbs water in your colon and prevents your stools from becoming hard and difficult to move through your colon.

Enzymes that digest your food come from fresh produce and from within your body. If you eat mostly processed foods, you will be using up your enzymes. When you are low on body enzymes, you will decrease your ability to digest foods. This will cause poor digestion, which creates acid wastes that your liver has to deal with.

Detoxifying Your Liver

Your liver needs plenty of fruits and vegetables every day, to detoxify. This produce has the fiber, nutrients, and antioxidants that your liver uses, to cleanse itself and other body organs.

Your liver also needs to see a reduction in the consumption of bad fatty acids, such as hydrogenated and partial hydrogenated oil found in all junk food. Hydrogenated oils are deadly and lead to cardiovascular diseases.

Liver Morning Drink

Using a hand juicer, you can press the juice out of 3 grapefruits and 3 lemons. Drink this right away. This drink will help to detoxify your liver and neutralize free some of its free radicals.

Power up this juice grapefruit-lemon drink by adding the following:

- 2 cloves of garlic and some ginger finely grated

- Add 2 tbsp. (30 ml) of cold pressed flax oil. The Omega 3 fatty acids in flax help balance the bile levels produced by the liver. Then drink this combination.

If you like you can make a tea of,

- Juice of one lemon

- 2-3 inches of chopped ginger

Now boil some water and add the chopped ginger for 5 minute. Wait for it to cool a bit, and then add the lemon. Drink this every morning, during your liver cleanse week, and you can also do this on other weeks that call for a herbal tea drink.

Herbs for Your Liver

- Milk Thistle (silymarin) - is one of the best herbs to help rejuvenate, protect, repair your liver. Standardized 80 percent silymarin is recommended for pills.

- Dandelion – improves liver function and stimulates the flow of bile into the gallbladder.

- Burdock root – purifies blood and stimulates bile flow from the liver. It helps to rebuild damaged liver cells.

- Artichoke (cynarin) – assists in bile production and flow and can help prevent gallstones. .

- Turmeric (curcumin) – reduces liver inflammation. You can empty turmeric capsules into heated milk or coconut oil and drink it. It makes the turmeric more bio-available.

These are the herbs to use for liver detoxifying and rebuilding. Mix these herbs together and make a tea. Then, drink two times a day.

Foods That Your Liver Loves

- Use these foods daily in your diet.

- Garlic – will activate your liver enzymes and flush out toxins

- Grapefruit – will help cleanse your liver of toxins.

- Beets and carrots – stimulate and improve liver function.

- Green Tea – has plenty of antioxidants to assist in liver function.

- Leafy Green Vegetables – help in cleansing your liver. It's the chlorophyll in the green that absorbs blood toxins

- Avocados – help the body produce glutathione, which neutralized free radicals.

- Apple – help your digestion system, which in turn helps lessen toxins that reach your liver.

- Whole Grains – like brown rice and red rice, contain nutrients that improve your liver fat metabolism and liver function and congestion.

- Cruciferous Vegetables and Cabbage – like broccoli, cabbage, and cauliflower improve liver enzymes that flush out toxins.

- Walnuts – support liver cleansing.

Good Oils

The good oils are omega-3, omega-6, fish oil, and flax seed oil, which are easily digested. You need to balance omega-3 to omega-6, by eating more omega -3 than omega-6. Eating excess omega-6 produces inflammatory prostaglandins that are involved in acne breakouts.

Olive oil has more omega-6 than omega-3, so use less of this oil. Most people use large quantities of olive oil, and this puts them out of balance with omega-3.

Flaxseed Oil

Flaxseed oil has more omega-3 than omega-6 that is why it has become a popular oil to use.

Here are other foods to eat for more omega-3 oil:

Flaxseed meal, plain flaxseed, **walnuts**, pumpkin seeds, brazil nuts, sesame seeds, avocados, kale spinach mustard greens, wheat germ oil, **salmon**, mackerel, halibut, sardines, anchovies, albacore tuna, **kidney beans**, navy beans.

Do not use olive oil for cooking. The heat oxidizes this oil, creating free radicals that will harm your body. In addition, do not fry fish, since the omega-3 will be damage and be of no value to your health.

The best oil to cook with is coconut oil. This oil can withstand high cooking temperatures before it decomposes.

Chapter Summary

Here again, the best way to cleanse your liver is to **Use Dr. Schulze's Liver Cleanse.**

Your **liver is the main organ** that controls how toxins will be detoxified and how they will be disposed of. It is also involved in balancing hormones and routing them to the right locations. You will want to have the best working liver, so that excess toxic material is eliminated properly and not through your skin.

Use your **liver diet with lots of fiber**, so that hormones are not reabsorbed back into your blood, from your colon.

Fruits and vegetables are the food your liver needs to detoxify. When you avoid eating hydrogenated junk food, you give your liver a chance to get well. Your liver loves the essential fatty acids and routes them to where they are needed to reduce inflammation.

Create a **grapefruit-lemon drink** with ginger and flax seed oil.

A simple but effective **liver cleansing drink** comes from a tea made from lemon and ginger.

Chapter 18: How Sleep And Stress Affect Acne

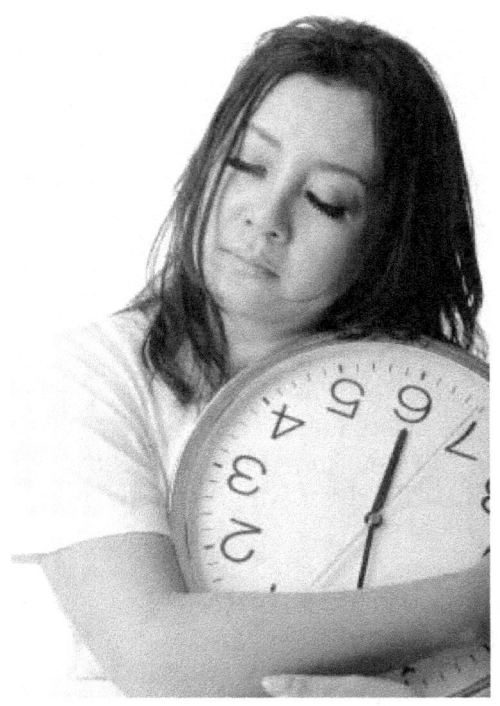

Chinese Medicine

In Chinese's medicine, each organ has an emotion associated with it. Your liver is associated with anger. If you harbor anger for a long time, this leads to an imbalance in your liver. If your liver is not balanced, then it can lead you to have anger. It's a cycle that can feed on itself.

When you have an imbalance in your liver, this can lead to acne or skin blemishes.

Anger

If you are angry with someone, you need to find a way to resolve it or get past this. Keeping your anger for long periods or maintaining high levels of anger or hatred, can affect your liver and result in illness and disease.

Anger can cause the lack of appetite, diarrhea, or indigestion. Suppressed anger can result in depression or menstrual disorders.

Studies have found that people who had high levels of hostility towards others have decreased immunity. A low immunity opens you up to skin blemishes, a variety of disease, and an increase in pathogen.

Fear and Letting Go

Your kidneys are associated with fear. When some people experience a lot of fear, their bladder becomes uncontrollable, and they urinate. Children may wet the bed, when they are fearful.

Excess worry about life situations or problems can also weaken your kidneys.

Your kidneys and bladder are also related to "letting go of negative emotions." Since your kidneys functions to remove un-needed body substances, it also works on eliminating bad emotions or keeping good emotions. Your kidneys have to balance everything that your body needs to keep healthy and to let go of that which is not.

Your kidneys also works hard, to keep your blood acid-alkaline balanced. You can see that keeping your kidneys working properly will improve your skin's health.

Past Emotions

Usually, it is difficult to deal with the emotions that affect your liver, kidney, and bladder. These emotions are normally suppressed feeling, from your childhood or past that were never resolved and have been triggered by present interaction with other persons. Past suppressed emotions are a major force in the formation illness and acne.

In his book called, Why You Get Sick How You Get Well, 1996, Dr. Arthur Janov says that all sickness starts in your mind. In his years of practicing psychotherapy at The Primal Institute in Los Angeles, CA, he discovered how past traumatic experience creates illness. Once the traumatic experience is relieved, the illness disappeared.

If you have acne, there are always some underlying emotions and feelings that are being expressed by your acne. Look into yourself and try to see what you are saying with your acne.

Acne can have some representation from repressed traumas that you have experienced as a child. Acne can be an expression of those traumas, trying to burst out. Your body has a defense mechanism that holds back and buries past traumas.

Some effort has to be made on your part, to connect and release these traumas. Otherwise, as you clear your face, these suppressed traumas can move to some other part of your body, where they will be unseen and destroy tissue and body functions.

All past suppressed trauma that you have experienced has a representation in the body, internally or externally. This representation can be an internal body weakness or disease.
Or, it can be topical condition like acne, boils, rashes, eczema, or psoriasis.

Your body protects you from early trauma that could have overwhelmed you, causing death or mental breakdown. It does this by suppressing the pain associated with the trauma. But, this suppressed pain is typically expressed by your body through distortions in your health, appearance or personality.

Daily Triggers

Past suppressed trauma remains hidden in your memory and throughout your body. The pain and suffering that you endured in the past is typically disconnected from your consciousness. This pain is usually triggered and brought into your consciousness by words, situations or events that occur in your present day's activities.

When your past pain is brought to consciousness, you will associate this pain with the interaction you are having with people in the present and not with past traumatic events.
This is how you can become angry, hurt, or depressed more than what the present events call for.

Studies have shown that people with acne tend to experience more anger, depression, anxiety, and suicidal feeling than those that do not have acne.

If you find that you over react to various present day situations, you may want to consider working with some good therapists.

Psychological Therapy

Psychological therapy may be of help in resolving anger and fear. Finding the right psychological process can be difficult, so if you have many emotional issues, this is the first place to start.

Tapes

Using hypnosis, affirmations, positive thinking, holosync tapes or hemisync tapes, or paraliminal tape, can be some help, but it is not a cure. These methods usually lead to continually suppression of your emotions, rather than providing a sort of cure. However, in combination with therapy, these tapes can be helpful and give you a way to relax and reduce simple stress.

Meditation

Meditation is an excellent way to deal with stress, anger, and fear. Here is a site where you can get some of the latest meditation tapes. (see resource section)

Herbs

Here are some herbs that you can use to relax you and to reduce the tension in your body.

Chamomile

Chamomile is sedative that can be used for mild anxiety or nervousness. This is an herb that can also benefit the health of your liver and lungs.

Kava Kava

Kava Kava is an excellent herb for calming moderate anxiety, stress, and insomnia. Do no use this, if you are on medication, drink alcohol, or have liver problems. Always test out an herb to see what your reaction will be, when you take it.

Hops

Hops is another herb that is great for stress, insomnia, and nervousness. In addition, hops can lower your body's acid level. It has also been found to be good for skin disorders, like acne.

Passionflower

Passionflower is another herb that is good for reducing muscle tension and reducing insomnia.

Valerian Root

Valerian root is good for insomnia, but is also good for anxiety, by reducing mental and physical tension.

Lavender

Lavender is effective in decreasing anxiety and promoting relaxation. It is also a powerful anti-bacterial and can work to balance hormones.

Licorice Root

Licorice root can help you during stressful times. It also helps to normalize your blood sugar levels.

Using These Herbs

The best way to use these herbs is to buy them in half or one oz. packets. Then, mix three or four of them in a one to one mixture. For example, one tablespoon of hops, one tablespoon of licorice root, one tablespoon of chamomile.

Boil this mixture, let it sit for 10 minutes, and drink it like a tea.

Food for Stress

Complex Carbohydrates

When you eat complex carbohydrates, like fruits, vegetables, and whole grains, you can reduce stress. Complex carbohydrates increase serotonin and provide the stimulus to feel good.

Oatmeal

Oatmeal is also known to reduce stress and at the same time raise your serotonin levels, thereby gives you a feeling of calmness.

Cabbage Juice

Drinking cabbage juice regularly can help you reduce nervousness, fear, depression, headaches, restlessness, and trembling, anxiety, and pessimistic views.

Use cabbage juice, when you are ill, since it improves your immune system and is a general tonic for the whole body.

Mix it with other juices, such as carrot juice, to make it tastier.

Exercise

Various exercises also will provide you stress relief, by releasing endorphins. Doing frequent exercises, will help you manage your anxiety and stress. Practicing Yoga has been found to be effective in reducing stress. But, this is true of the many other exercises you might do.

Sleep

Eight to nine hours of sleep are typically what most people need to maintain a healthy body and to help prevent acne. When you don't get the sleep, you need, your body produces excess hormones to compensate for this.

During the night, your body is busy digestion, repairing, rebuilding, and detoxifying your body. As you sleep, every hour each organ has it turn in rejuvenating and detoxifying itself.

It's best to get to bed early and get the sleep your body needs. When you toss and turn and wake frequently at night, you are not getting the rest you need.

Ways to Get More Sleep.

For Men

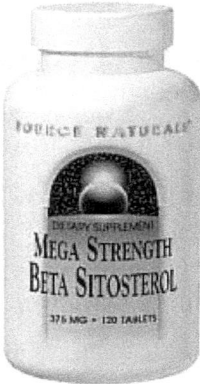

If you get up at night to urinate 2-3 times or wake up early in the morning to do this, you, mostly likely, have an enlarged prostrate. An enlarged prostrate will narrow your urinary track and not allow you to release all your urine from your bladder at one time. The result is you have to urinate frequently, during the night.

This will certainly have an impact on getting a good night sleep. Here is a supplement, **Mega Strength Beta Sitosterol**, that will help your eliminate frequent night urination and reduce weak and trickling urine.

Melatonin

Melatonin is a hormone released by your Pinal gland. As the day gets darker, your Pinal gland starts to release melatonin. If you wake up at night and can't get to sleep again or wake up too early, take 2-4 mg of melatonin before you get to bed.

Experiment with the dose to figure out what is best for you. You can purchase melatonin in sublingual or time release pills. Sublingual melatonin works fast and is easier to use.

Psychological Nutrients

The nutrients that are needed for psychological issues are,
- Zinc

- Folic acid
- Selenium
- Chromium
- Omega-3
- Digestive enzymes
- Anti-oxidants
- 5 HTP

5 HTP Supplements

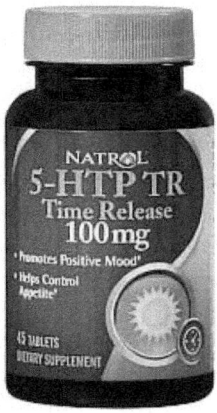

If you are plagued with depression, obesity, and craving carbohydrates, the supplement to take is **5 HTP.** You want to make sure that you have some of these supplements in your diet.

Chapter Summary

Anger and fear are detrimental to your health. These emotions create acid, which takes minerals to neutralize them. Anger is a **liver emotion,** and an excess of this emotion can affect the health of your liver.

Fear is related to your kidneys. When you experience a lot of fear, your kidneys become weak and are unable to balance your blood minerals and toxins properly.

Past traumatic experiences that you might have contribute to your wellbeing. This trauma is well represented in your body, by your life opinions, your physical appearance, and your overall health.

Past trauma embeds itself in your body, creating distortion in your body functions. These distortions lead to an expression of diseases, such as acne, psoriasis, eczema, cardiovascular conditions, and array other diseases.

If you need **psychological therapy**, then you should seek it to reduce the stress on your liver, kidneys, and elimination channels. You can use hemi sync, paraliminal, or meditation tapes to give you some stress relief. In addition, you can also drink herbs to relax you. Exercise is another form of stress relief.

You need **the best sleep** you can get. This will help you regenerate your body. One of the best ways to get deep sleep is to use melatonin. Use two to four mg each night. Melatonin is a hormone and anti-oxidant for your body and brain.

For men with frequent night urination issues, take Mega Strength Beta Sitosterol or another beta sitosterol product.

Look over the list of **psychological nutrients** that you need to take. Many of these nutrients are already required to help control acne.

Consider that **many of your thoughts are wrong** and what you think you should do, you should not. Consider doing the opposite of what you think you should. This type of thinking can bring on a new perspective to your life and start to unravel what you think is right.

Chapter 19: Acne Herbal Remedies

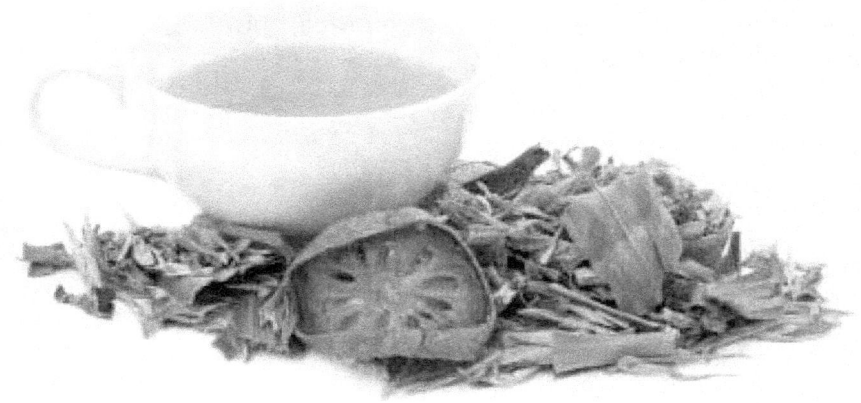

Herbal Teas for Acne

You will find many health stores that sell loose herbs. If you don't have such a store in your city, go to the Internet to buy from ½ oz to 1 once of each herb. Then mix the appropriate herbs together, based on the formulas listed below.

Using herbal mixtures can sometimes increase your acne activity temporarily. Don't panic, since herbs are a powerful way to cleanse your blood and start the acne healing process.

Mix a tea, which contains the following herbs,
- Figwort 1 ounce

- Turkey corn 1 ounce

- Echinacea 1 ounce

- Thuja 1 ounce

- Yellow dock 1 ounce

- Arctium lappa ½ ounce
- Iris versicolor ½ ounce

You can also make a tea using any one of the following herbs. You can also mix 3 to 4 of these herbs, to make your own special herbal tea. Mix them with equal amounts. Drink the tea throughout the day.

- Burdock
- Dandelion
- Echinacea
- Fragrant valerian
- Goldenseal
- Ivy
- Marshmallow root
- Purslane
- Watercress
- Wild strawberry leaves
- Yarrow root
- Eucalyptus
- Oregon grape root
- Thai sweet and holy basil oil

You can sometimes find premixed herbal teas that are for acne at your favorite health-food store. Check their content to make sure they have some of the herbs listed above.

Herbal Extracts

Herbal extracts are herb made in an alcoholic solvent or in a non-alcoholic solvent. Here's an herbal extract that is designed for acne. Its main function is to improve the liver function, purify the blood, reduce acne inflammation, and fight acne bacterial infections.

This herbal extract is a liquid and is taken in water or as drops into your mouth. You will be able to find this mixture on the Internet.

Burdock-Sarsaparilla Compound - contains the following herbs.

- Burdock mature seed - helps to purify the liver, balance hormones, neutralizes acid, is anti-inflammatory, and purifies the blood.
- Jamaican sarsaparilla root – helps scaling skin, is blood purifying, reduces itching, and helps balance hormones
- Nettle mature seed – is anti-inflammatory for the skin, neutralizes acid waste with its high mineral content
- Yellow dock root – rich in iron and works to improve liver function, helps build good blood, purifies blood and lymphatic liquid, increases bile, and reduces constipation.
- Spilanthes flowing herb – improves immunity to fight bacterial infections on the skin.
- Sassafras root bark – blood cleansing, and anti-inflammatory for the skin,

This is excellent herbal remedy and is not very expensive. If you can find it at a health-food store, it should cost around $12.00 or less. If not, then you can order it on the Internet and pay around $20.00, shipping included.

Here's how to take this herbal extract.

Take 30 – 35 drops in water three times a day. Take it for six days, then let your body rest and start again after the seventh day.

Foot Spa

If you have a foot spa, this is your chance to use it, for acne. It's a pleasant and convenient way, to get herbal nutrition into your body. The soles of your feet allow nutrients to get into your blood stream easily.

When you use a heated footbath, veins in your feet start to expand. Over a period of 15-20 minute, the warm water affects your entire vascular (blood) system, and you get improved blood circulation.

By adding herbs to your hot water, minerals and other phytochemicals from the herbs enter the soles of your feet and into your blood stream.

Herbs for a Footbath or Tea

This herbal combination was taken and modified slightly from a book written by Daniel B. Mowrey, Ph.D., called The Scientific Validation of Herbal Medicine, 1986. In his book Mowrey says,

"This (herbal) blend attacks external skin disorders from within, purifying the blood, carrying away waste, reinforcing the blood's ability to ward off infectious agents."

You can use 1 or more in your footbath and to drink as a tea.

Just buy the herbs you want to use and mix them in equal parts. You can pick two or three herbs and get the benefits listed below.

The herbal combination to use is,

- Dandelion root – purifies blood and improves liver function.
- Yellow dock root – purifies blood, helps liver, is anti-bacterial.
- Saraparilla root – has antibiotic action, promotes waste elimination through urine and sweating.
- Echinacea – increases immunity and promotes skin healing.
- Licorice – protects the liver, so that it can detoxify the blood better.
- Kelp – provides minerals and vitamins and binds heavy metals that are bad for your health.
- Chaparral – is anti-microbial, making it effective against pathogens.
- Garlic – is anti-parasitic – use chopped cloves.
- Ginger – helps circulate blood – use chopped ginger.

Buy half an ounce of each herb you like and mix them.
Here's how to do the herbal footbath,

- Place 2 tbsp of the herbal mix into a pot with 1 ½ cups of water
- Boil the water with herbs – use a glass, porcelain, or stainless steel container
- After the water starts to boil, pull the container of the stove

- Let the tea sit for 15-30 minutes. The longer the tea sits the stronger the tea and its effects
- Prepare your foot spa with water and heat
- Strain the tea to remove leaves and roots
- Pour tea into your foot spa
- Place your feet in hot water as high as you can stand for 15 – 30 minutes. Careful not burn your feet. Start the bubbler, if you have one.

Chapter Summary

Herbal teas have the power to help you recover your health. They are not used as much as they were in the past. For acne, herbal teas make a lot of sense. They provide the water to flush out toxins. They are filled with nutrients and anti-oxidants that prevent diseases and improve body functions.

You can **mix your own teas** from a variety of loose herbs. A list of herbs has been given, in this chapter to do just this. Make an herbal tea and use it every day, for a week, and then make a different one for the next week, to get the nutrients and benefits of different herbs.

You can make enough tea for two days, but you need to keep it in a thermos and refrigerator.

Herbal extracts are also good to use, since you can place them in water or juice and drink them right away.

You can use a **foot spa**, if you have one and put many of the herbs into the spa listed in this chapter. Choose any of the herbs you want, for the benefits that they give.

Chapter 20: Supplements To Take For Acne

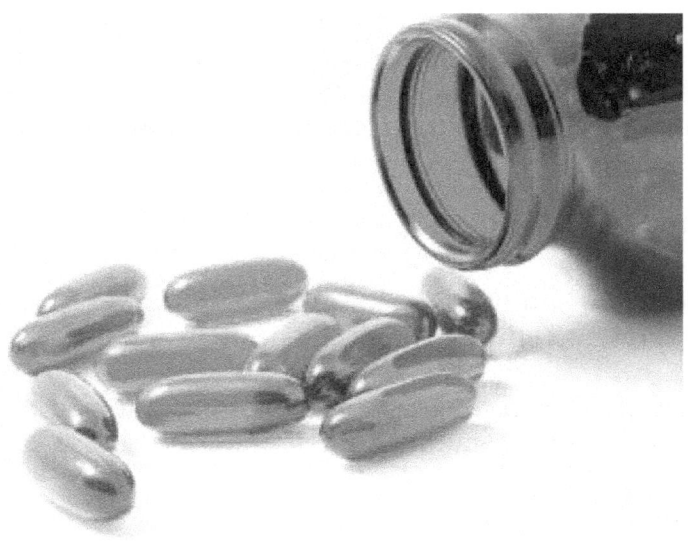

Vitamins

Here are some of the vitamins and minerals you should be taking to help you get rid of acne.

- Vitamin D3 – 3000 to 4500 IU in the morning and night for a total of 6000 to 9000 IU. Do not excess more than 10,000 IU without taking vitamin K.
- B6, 25 – 150 mg in a B vitamin complex
- B5 pantothenic acid, 500 – 1000 mg per day
- Vitamin A (water soluble), 25,000 to 30,000 IU – take just before meals. Taking more than 50,000 IU requires a Doctors approval.
- Vitamin C, buffered 1000mg three times a day

- Vitamin E, 400 IU, two times a day before meals for a total of 800 IU a day.

A word of caution: Do not take more than 50,000 IUs of vitamin A, since it can be toxic at higher levels. If you experience any symptoms with 50,000 IUs of vitamin A, then you should back off to 25,000 units. Eating vegetables that have high levels of beta carotene can help you get the vitamin A that your body needs.

Minerals

Here are some of the minerals you should be taking to help control and eliminate acne.

Use a calcium-magnesium mixture. Take a tablet after each meal. Take the quantity listed under the label.

Chromium

Zinc

Vitamin C

Vitamin E

Vitamin B

MSM

Beta Carotene

Saw Palmetto

Mineral electrolytes

Take Zinc gluconate 25 – 60 mg a day **(zinc is one of the most important nutrients to add to your diet.)** Zinc works to reduce the male sex hormone dihyrdrotestosterone (DHT), which in excess will produce acne. Do not take over 100 mg, unless you consult with a Doctor.

Word of Caution: After you have gained relief from acne, you can discontinue the use of high doses of the supplements listed above and get back to your normal supplementation program.

Special Supplements to Take

There are seven special supplements that you should consider taking, to improve your overall health for now and for the future. These supplements will improve your immune system and help to clear and prevent future acne. Look over these supplements and take the one or ones that you feel will give you the most benefits, for your health. Some of these supplements may become part of your overall health program, when you finish this acne system.

- Electrolyte Minerals
- Digestive or systemic enzymes
- Flax Seed Oil
- Lecithin
- Chlorophyll and Lemon
- Vitamin D3

Electrolyte Minerals

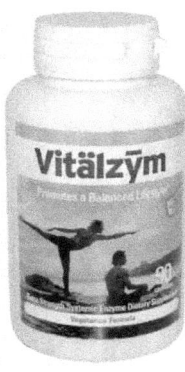

The skin needs plenty of minerals. You can use a mineral supplement to get them. Here is an excellent liquid mineral to use - **Crystalloid Electrolytes**.

Use this supplement in your juices Systemic Enzymes.

If you have scars or pockmarks that have recently occurred from acne, you may be able to clear them, by using a **product called Vitalzym**.

You're not going to hear this from your doctor or dermatologist, but systemic enzymes, such as serapeptase, found in Vitalzym capsules, can remove excess fibrin, which makes up scar tissue.

Systemic enzymes have a different function from digestive enzymes. Systemic enzymes work in your body organs, tissue, skin, and joints to remove excess fibrin. Fibrin accumulates when you have surgical scars or internal injuries, which helps to repairs such areas.

Take systemic capsules between meals

Digestive Enzymes

Digestive enzymes are used to help you digest the food you eat. If you eat mostly processed foods, these foods don't have digestive enzymes to help digest themselves. Your body has to use up its own digestive enzymes.

If you have been eating processed food for years and little raw live food, your digestive enzyme supply will diminish, and you will not digest food as good as when you were younger.

Take digestive enzymes with every meal.

This will reduce the amount of undigested food that gets into your colon, which forms toxic acids.

Flax Seed Oil

Flax seed oil has an anti-inflammatory effect on the body and on skin diseases. It will help to reduce or relieve the inflammation of your acne. This is a good fat and provides you with more omega-3 than omega-6.

Take one tablespoon or more a day. This can be done easily, when you add it to salads or other food that are already cooked.

Lecithin

Lecithin is made from soybeans and is found in health-food stores in yellow granules. It is an emulsifier, which is a substance that helps fats and nonfat to mixed and stay together, without separating.

In your blood, it keeps the fats from forming large globes, which can create problems, if your arteries are narrow. Lecithin also has many other benefits such as,

- Improving digestion and absorption of essential fatty acids (omega-3 and omega-6)
- Improving skin problems
- Improving memory
- Lowering cholesterol

Add 1-2 tablespoons of lecithin granules to your smoothies.

Add one or two teaspoons of granules to your soups or other liquid food.

Sprinkle one teaspoon of granules on your fresh salads.

Chlorophyll and Lemon

Here is something you should drink every day during the week.

It's a drink that combines liquid chlorophyll and one lemon juice.

Chlorophyll is one of the best ways to detoxify your colon fast. It is an antioxidant, anti-inflammatory, anti-microbial agent, and absorber of heavy metals in your colon. It also helps to improve your hemoglobin count, which will then give you more oxygen.

You cannot overdose on chlorophyll liquid that is why you can use 2 ounces or more and the juice from one lemon in an eight oz glass of water. Chlorophyll is one of the benefits you get when you eat dark-green vegetables. Vitex, Chasteberry for Hormonal Balance

Vitex is a hormonal tonic, for women that stimulate and normalize your pituitary gland. It is your pituitary gland that balances the amount of progesterone and estrogen in your body.

When estrogen and progesterone get out of balance, as they do during menstruation, acne can be created. Vitex helps to increase progesterone and decrease estrogen during menstruation.

Because Vitex helps to support and feed the endocrine system, it can be use anytime, but is quite useful during menstruation. This herb can be used as a tea, capsule, or extract (alcohol extract or tincture)

As a tincture use 30 to 50 drops, three times a day.

Since Vitex is a slow-acting herb, use it daily and add it to your long term supplement use.

It is a safe herb. However, a few people may exhibit minor side effects, such as nausea, headache, stomach upset, and skin rashes. Check with your doctor for use, when pregnant or when depressed.

Not recommend for men.

Female Formula by Dr. Schulze

Dr. Schulze has done it again, by preparing a **female herbal formula extract.** It contains some of the better-known herbs that help your pituitary, hypothalamus and ovaries communicate to create hormonal balance.

It contains dong quai, wild yam, chaste tree, licorice root, hops flowers, and damiana leaf. This combination of herbs can help even out the hormones needed to regulate menopause, PMS, menstrual irregularity, and infertility. If your hormones are unbalanced for other reasons, this herbal formula is what you need.

Licorice for Hormonal balance

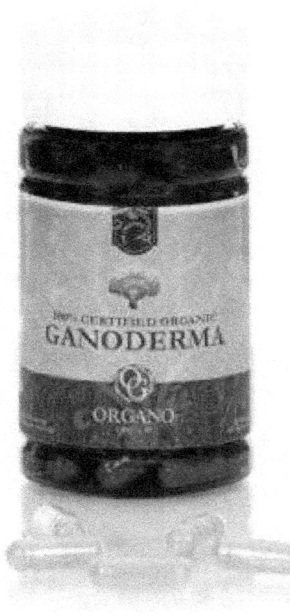

Licorice herb is frequently used for hormonal problems, since it affects androgen metabolism. It blocks the enzymes that are involved in the creation of androgens andestrogens. Excess androgens and estrogens are a key in forming acne.

But, more important is that licorice reduces the conversion of testosterone into DHT, a hormone that is associated with acne production.

Ganoderma Lucidum, Reishi Mushrooms Gandoerma lucidum or Reishi is a mushroom found in East Asia, which suppresses the conversion of testosterone to DHT.

Ganderma contains germanium and other minerals that help your body detoxify, by removing toxins from your body and cleansing your liver and blood. The detoxification occurs through your skin, which causes more acne as you start to use it. When detoxification is complete, Ganderma stops producing acne.

Thyroid Supplement

Your thyroid gland needs a high level of trace minerals to produce the thyroid hormone, T4 and to convert it to the active T3 hormone. **The minerals you want are selenium, zinc, manganese, and iodine**. When you lack these minerals, your thyroid will be sluggish, and you will have a low metabolism or hypothyroidism. Low metabolism will show up as a low temperature in your underarm thyroid morning test. This will lead to lack of energy, focus, and craving for sugar and junk food.

Here is a product called Selenomune that contains all the trace minerals and more than you need to improve your thyroid and immune function.

Chapter Summary

There are a variety of **basic supplements** that should take during this acne program. When the program is over, you don't have to take so many supplements, because you will be eating better and a lot of the minerals, vitamins, and nutrients will come from your food.
The **important vitamins** to take in the beginning of this program are vitamin D3, A C, E, B100 complex, zinc, and selenium.

For **minerals** take calcium, magnesium and chromium.

There are many different nutritional supplements to use. **Chlorophyll** is a powerful body detoxifier and should always be part of your regular health program.

Digestive enzymes are also critical to ensure good digestion. A good systemic enzyme will work to help minimize acne scars. Of course, if your scars are deep, and you have had them for a long time, these enzymes may not work or may take a long time to work.

Lecithin granules help you digest fats. They also improve your skin appearance. Use 1-2 tablespoons in your smoothies, salads, or food.

Chapter 21: Best Essential Fatty Acids

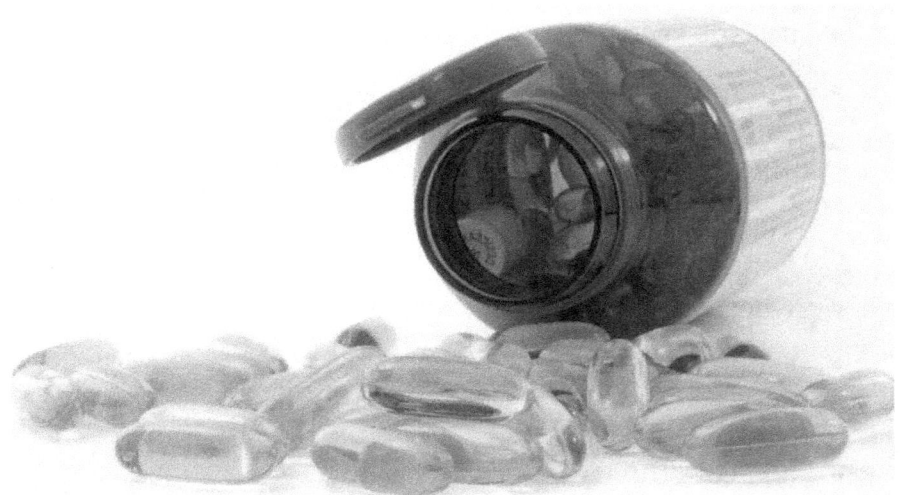

Getting Your Fatty Acids

Getting sufficient essential fatty acids is of prime importance in clearing acne. It's these fatty acids that help to control the production of androgens, which causes excess sebum oil to clog your hair follicles and create acne.

The three most important fatty acids you need every day are omega-3, omega-6, and omega-9. You need two to three times more omega-6 than omega-3. Most people eat 8 to 12 times more omega-6 than omega-3. This causes an imbalance in the omegas and leads to body inflammation.

- Use flax seed oil (omega-3 oil) and olive oil (omega-6 oil) in your salad.

- The other oil that is even better for you is called

monounsaturated fatty acid, omega-9. This oil is found in avocados and in small amounts in most oils.

You can get omega-3 oil from,

- avocados

- sesame seeds

- pumpkin seeds

- walnuts

- dark leafy green vegetables (spinach, mustard greens, kale)

- wheat germ oil

- salmon

- sardines

- albacore tuna

You can take two to three tablespoon of flax seed oil each day. This will give you the amount of omega-3 oil that your body needs. You can add this oil to your morning cereal, ready to eat soups, smoothies, salads and other liquid foods. Never cook or heat flax seed oil, since it oxidizes quickly and becomes rancid.

You can get omega-6 oil from,

- Flaxseed oil

- Flaxseeds

- grape seed oil

- pistachio nuts

- olives

- olive oil

- sunflower seeds

- chicken

- evening primrose oil

- pumpkin seeds

- pine nuts

Taking 2-3 tablespoons of omega-6 oil a day will give you the amount of this oil that your body needs. You can add olive oil and other oils into your salad with the flax seed oil.
You can get omega-9 oil from,

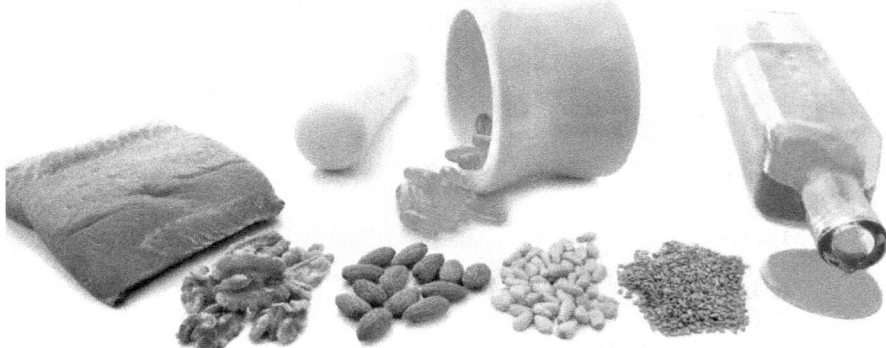

- Olive oil

- Avocados

- Peanuts

- Cashews

- Almonds

- Olives

- sesame oil

- pecans

- pistachio nuts

Taking around 1 ½ tablespoon of olive oil per day will give you the omega-9 oil that your body needs.
Other oils that are good for your skin are,

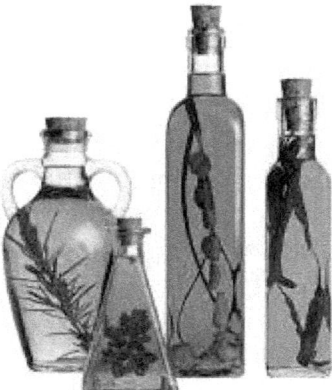

- Apricot kernel oil
- Coconut oil
- Peanut oil
- Almond oil
- Sesame oil
- Sunflower oil
- Wheat germ oil

Use these oils on salads; add a tablespoon to juice, or to a smoothie. Use only coconut oil for cooking.

Fish Oils

In addition to supplying your diet with omega-3 and omega-6 oils, you need to supplement your diet with fish oils. Fish oil contains EPA and DHA fatty acids.

Normally, enzymes in your body break down omega-6 into these fatty acids,
- Dihomo-gamma-linolenic acid (DGLA)

- Arachidonic Acid (AA)

- Eicosapentaenoic Acid (EPA)

- Docosahexaenoic Acid (DHA)

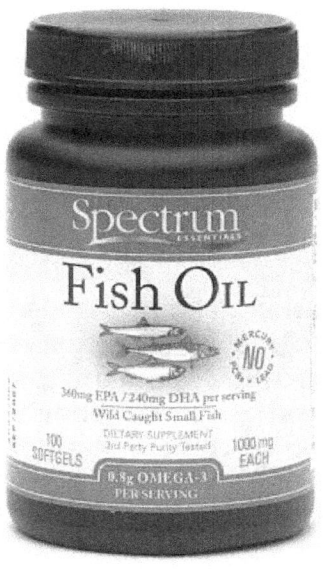

Of course eating salmon, halibut, and mackerel twice a week will be a plus in providing your body with more EPA and DHA.

Here is an excellent fish oil product. Omega-3 Norwegian Fish Oil, by Spectrum Essentials

Two capsules contain,
EPA – 360mg

DHA – 240mg

Omega-3 – 892mg

Stearic Lauric Palmitic Acids - 508 mg

Using the Omega-3 Norwegian Fish Oil or other fish oil is critical in getting relief from acne, so take two capsules per meal.
Eat cold-water fish at least twice a week to provide EPA and DHA to your diet

Daily Essential Fatty Acid Requirements

Here are the daily supplementation requirements for the omega fatty acids.

- 3000 mg of linoleic – omega-6 fatty acid

- 1800 mg of linolenic – omega-3 fatty acid

GLA Sources

GLA provides your skin with many benefits such as, forming the structure of skin cell membranes, keeping your skin lubricated with oil and water, and protecting it from toxic matter.

There are different sources for supplementing with GLA.
- Borage Oil
- Primrose Oil

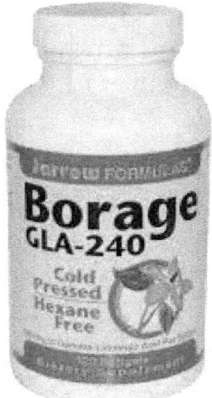

These two oils are high in GLA with Borage oil being the highest. In addition, they also contain Omega-6 oil.

The important information to know here is, GLA has the ability to block the activity of male hormones, androgens, which in an excess cause an over production of sebum oil.

These hormones are in both males and females.

GLA also provides relief for other skin issues such as,
- Skin dryness
- Inflammation
- Pimple oozing
- Itching

Borage Oil

How to Use It

Take two 1000 mg of borage oil soft gels each day, with meals.

Borage oil can also be added to your acne cream by breaking open a soft gel capsule and mixing it into the cream. This will provide GLA directly onto your skin, where it is needed to control acne and other skin disorders.

Primrose Oil

Primrose oil is another source of GLA.

Take 1000 mg soft gel capsule four times a day with a meal or snack.

Chapter Summary

Because **essential fatty acids** are critical for the success of this acne program, you need to know where to get them. The fatty acids are omega-3, 6, and 9 oils. Use **flaxseed oil** in your food and supplement with **fish oil**. Look over the ingredients of the Omega-3 Norwegian Fish Oil.
There are **certain foods** like avocados, nuts and seeds, and green leafy vegetables that have fatty acids. You should eat as much of this food, as possible. Using a **variety of oils** in your food, can give you the omegas you need.

There are **daily essential fatty acid requirements,** and you will find that they are more than what you thought. You need a lot of omega fatty acids in your body, to keep you healthy and to control acne inflammation.

Chapter 22: Facial Using Benzoyl Peroxide

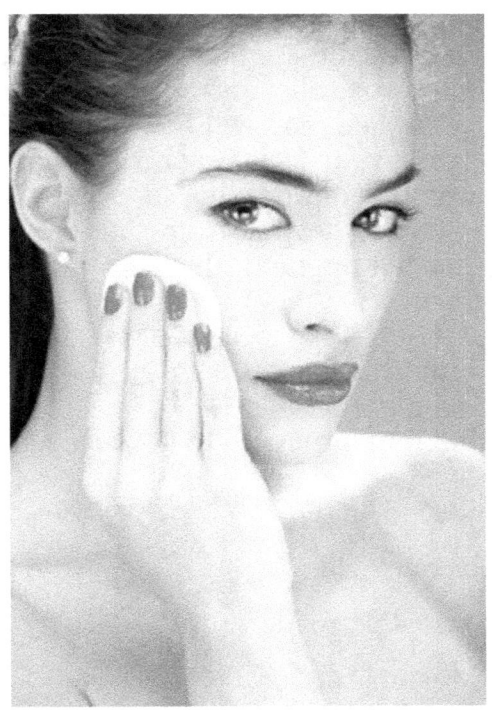

Purpose of This Chapter

In this chapter, you have a step by step facial cleansing method, using salicylic acid, glycolic acid, and benzoyl peroxide. This is a proven technique for getting rid of acne on your face. However, this alone will not get rid of acne for good.

Facial Cleansing Method

You will start doing facials every day during the second week of this acne program. There are three different facials that you will be using.

Use this facial cleansing method in conjunction with internal cleansing, to clean up your internal organs.

By combining both methods, you are attacking your acne from the inside, which gives you long term acne curing and from the outside, which gives you relief and curing of your present acne. In this cleansing method, you will be working directly on your skin, to start healing your facial blemishes that you now have. Follow the instructions carefully, so that you get the best results. If you start to deviate from the instructions, you go against a time-tested method that has produced excellent results for others.

What You Need for This Facial Cleanse

Here are the different products that you need for this facial cleanse.

- Using Salicylic Acid

- Using Glycolic Acid

- Using Benzoyl peroxide

- Using a Moisturizer

- Scotty's Acne Cream

- Herbs–green tea non-caffeinated

- fresh ginger, oregano leaf

- Lemons

- Vitamin E

- Aloe Vera

- glycerin soap

- Pot or facial steamer for herbs

- towel

Staring Your Facial Cleansing

The first step is to start boiling 5 cups or more of water. Put green tea, plenty of pieces of ginger, and a heaping tablespoon of oregano leaf into a boiling pot of water.

Let water and herbs boil about 10 minutes.

As soon as the herbs are ready, wash your face with glycerin soap.

Place the hot pot with herbs on a surface that will not burn or spot. Place a towel over your head and move over the hot herb pot to steam your face.

Caution: Keep a safe distance away from the hot pot and steam, so that you don't burn your skin. Your skin will start to sweat as your pores open.

Breathe in deeply with your nose and exhale through your mouth, so that the steam can get into your lungs to get the herbal steam benefit.

Steam your face with these herbs for 6 minutes.

Now, take a cup and fill it with 1/2 hot tea and 1/2 water, to make it warm. Rinse your face with this warm tea three times Pat yourself dry with a towel. You are now ready to start the Salicylic Acid treatment.

NOTE: You will do this herbal steam cleanse for only two days.

Water Facial Steaming

After two days of using the herbal steaming, you will do a plain water steam, without herbs, for two days. So, you will be alternating with 2 days herbal steam and 2 day plain water steam.

Using Salicylic Acid

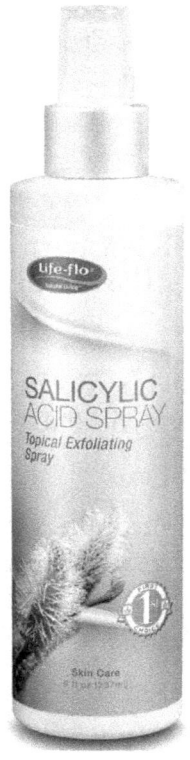

The second step is to **use Salicylic Acid**. When you use salicylic acid on your face, it serves to remove dead skin cells, and the dead follicle cells that combine with your sebum to plug up your pores, at the surface of your skin. It also helps reduce the bad bacteria that can accumulate on the surface of your skin and in your follicles.

Salicylic acid also provides an anti-inflammatory benefit by reducing the inflammation around your pores. This helps to open these pores slightly to allow salicylic acid to move deep into your pores to clean them out.

Buy a 2 % salicylic acid and no less. You can go to the Internet and search to this acid or go to your favorite drug store and ask for it. This product comes in pads or gel.

Applying the Salicylic Acid

This is how you apply the salicylic acid, and you will do this for two weeks, twice a day. You will do this one time in the morning and evening.

If you have acne in different parts of your face or body start with one area, then go to the next area.

- First, you splash warm water onto your face.

- Put about the size of a dime or more of salicylic acid on your hand.
- Mix a few drops of distilled water into salicylic acid. Make sure the two are mixed well. This dilutes the salicylic acid.
- In a circular movement, rub the salicylic acid and water mixture into the area that is covered with acne.
- Now, go to the next area that has acne, wet that area with water, then rub in the salicylic acid like before.
- Leave the salicylic acid on your face for about 5 minutes or for the time as instruction on the salicylic package.
- After 5 minutes, rinse the salicylic off with warm water and dry your face.

Using Glycolic Acid

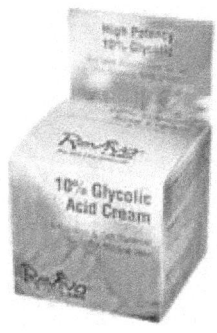

To unplug and dissolve your follicles of dead cells and sebum, which occur deep into your follicles, you need to use glycolic acid. It is this trapped mixture of dead cells and sebum that plug up your follicles that lead to an infected pimple.

Use an **8-10% Glycolic Acid** with no other active additives.

Glycolic acid is used immediately after you use salicylic acid, and you use it in just the same way. Let it stay on your skin for 5 minutes or as recommended on the container. Use Glycolic acid only once a day, in the morning.

Using Benzoyl Peroxide (BP) in the Evening

Now, for the next step in this facial cleanse, you will use Benzoyl Peroxide or BP. Using BP will stabilize your face more, since the first steps still leave the pores on your face inflamed, with pus, bacteria and excess sebum.

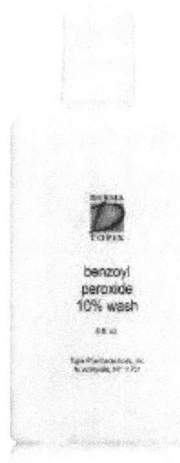

This pus and other material is way down into your pores or follicles, where it is hard to get to. If this pus is not removed, it will just continue to create the acne you are trying to get rid of.

Using BP allows you to move oxygen deep into your pores, where it acts as antibacterial, killing bacteria embedded deep into the pores.

First, you want to buy a **10% solution of Benzoyl Peroxide**.

Use BP in the evening after you use Salicylic Acid. Here's how to start.

Store your BP in the refrigerator and allow it to cool, before you use it.

Freeze some distilled water into ice cubes.

Take an ice cube and rub it across your acne infected area. Just get your skin cold and wet, but don't leave the ice cube too long on your face, otherwise you can burn your skin.

Place a few drops of BP on your palm of your hand or on a cold dish that was in the refrigerator. If you use your palm, cool it down with an ice cube and, then put a few drop of BP onto it.

Prepare and apply the BP just like you did with Salicylic acid. Add a drop of water to BP, mix it, and then rub it in a circular motion, onto your infected area.

After you have applied the BP, place cold packs from the refrigerator onto your infected area.

If you are working with two infected areas, then you need to apply a cold pack on each one. Get a thin cloth or paper towel to place between the cold pack and your facial skin, to prevent burning your skin from the cold pack. Use a thicker cloth, if your skin gets too cold.

Leave this cold pack on for 8-10 minutes. You may have to be lying down to keep the cold packs in position.

After the 8 - 10 minute cold pack, wipe your face off with a clean cloth and leave the BP residue on your face overnight. If the BP has a stinging effect, you may have to leave it on another day or when you get used to it.

After Using BP

Now, if after you using BP, you sense an excessive burning or itching, you can alternate the use of BP with Glycolic acid every other day. But use the Glycolic acid just as describe for the BP, ice and everything else.

If you just feel some tingling and no uncomfortable burning on your face, after BP, then you can use it every day.

There you have it. These three steps should help get rid of your acne in 5- 7 weeks or less.
But, you will only be using this cleansing for two weeks and after that, you will use the second cleansing method.

Using this method can get you started in cleaning out your pores.

Using a Moisturizer

Now, for the final step, you need to use a moisturizer every day after you have cleansed your skin in the morning with salicylic and glycolic acid.

The moisturizer will help to keep your skin healthy looking and resistant to the start of new acne.

Here's the type of moisturizer you need to use:
- Oil free

- Moisturizer with sun block of 30 or higher

Use a good **sun screen** each day, when completing the daily cleanses. This is to prevent infected pimples turning a dark color.

Use the moisturizer 2-3 times a day, if you feel
your skin is drying out, or if you are in the sun for long periods of time. You may want to renew your moisturizer, on your face, to get more sun block onto your skin.

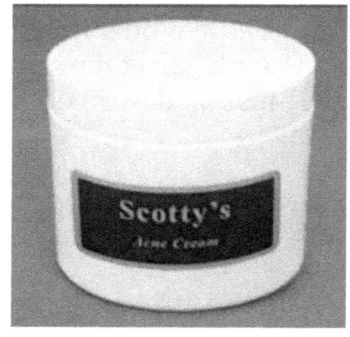

In addition to your moisturizer, you can use an acne cream called **Scotty's Acne Cream**. It's an excellent face cream you can use just before bedtime and during the day after
your cleansing. This cream contained all natural ingredients.

- It contains natural oils that rejuvenate the skin

- It contains minerals that help to reduce inflammation and rebuild the cell structure

- It contains nutrients that promoted skin regeneration and healing

You can put Scotty's cream first and then put your sunscreen. There you have it, a facial cleansing process that will help eliminate your acne, keep your skin clean, and reduce acne breakouts.

What to Do After This Acne Program Is Completed

First, continue using a moisturizing cream and Scotty's acne cream.

Using Scotty's Acne Cream

After you have washed your face, use a clean pad and massage Scotty's cream on your face and spread it all around.

These oils, in Scotty's, will seal your pores and hold the natural moisture on your skin and enhance the curing effects of the cream.

You can use this cream 2-3 times a day. It is best to use it after you have cleaned your face in the morning, and right before you go to bed.

You can use Scotty's' cream under your makeup or over your makeup. It will work either way. However, it will work better on a clean face.

You will notice that when you apply the cream, it will tingle in areas, without sores and may sting in open sores. This will pass and as it does, it should reduce the itchiness, of any sore.

Scotty's cream has allantoin, which will help to clear acne sores. The oils, vitamin A and E, and minerals in Scotty's will help to feed rebuild, and rejuvenate your skin. The minerals also help to neutralize the toxic acids that have contaminated and inflamed the pores.

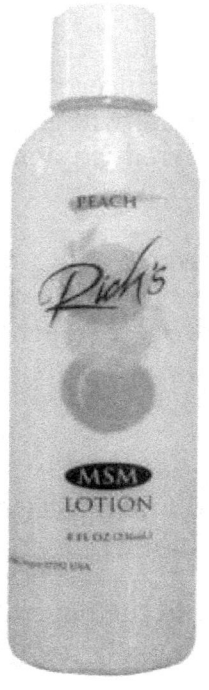

During cleansing and fasting, more acid waste may come out of your pores. This is why Scotty's cream will help you to reduce the inflammation and the spread of your acne.

MSM Fruit Medley Lotion

As a moisturizer, you can also use **Rich's MSM Lotion**, Fruit Medley, sold by richdistributng .com.

This is also a great cream because it has MSM in it. MSM is organic sulfur, and it will penetrate your skin and supply sulfur to the skin cells. Every cell in your body uses sulfur in its surround membrane.

Sulfur makes your cells stay healthy, by improving their permeability. It makes skin softer and flexible.

Tree Tea Oil

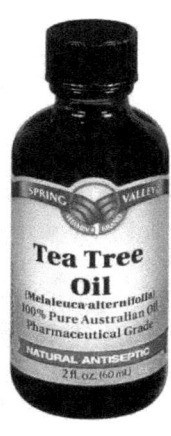

To make Scotty's cream even more powerful, you can add 5-10 drops of pure tree tea oil to a two-ounce container. You can experiment with the amount to add. You may want to add more drops to provide more tea tree oil for your face. But, do not use more than 15 drops.

Tree tea oil is effective in various skin disorders.

It acts as an antiseptic, antifungal, andantibacterial. This oil helps to bring oxygen to your skin cells, which kills bacteria and fungus and helps to repair damaged skin caused by acne.

Borage Oil

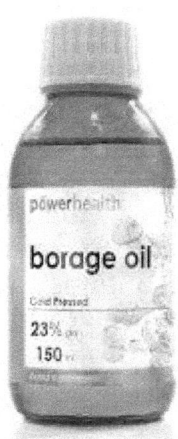

There is one more thing that you can add to Scotty's face cream that will boost its acne clearing power. This is borage oil. **Borage oil** contains EPA and DHA, which helps to control excessive hormones and over production of sebum.

It is the adrenal glands that produce streams of androgens during puberty. These large quantities of androgens help to activate bone growth and assist in bringing forth sexual maturity.

A side effect of these androgens is the release of excess oil from the oil glands near the hair follicle. This excess gives rise to,

- black heads
- white heads
- pimples
- cysts

So here's what you can do to make Scotty's face cream even more effective,

- Mix one or two capsules of Borage oil into Scotty's cream

- Do this by cutting the tip off of a Borage oil soft gel and squeezing the oil into the cream

Neptune Krill Oil (NKO)

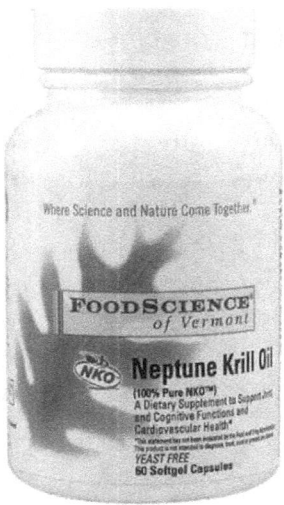

There is a new form of EPA and DHA that is available in a product called **Neptune Krill Oil (NKO)**

NKO is the new EPA and DHA product, which may be better to use than Borage Oil. NKO has the omega-3, EPA and DHA in the phospholipid form, which is easier for your cells to absorb compared with Borage oil. Borage oil contains the omega-3, EPA, and DHA in triglyceride form, which is more difficult for cells to absorb.

Also, NKO does not have to be refrigerated like Borage does. It can be kept in a cool place in your cabinets. However, it does cost more than Borage oil.

Word of Caution: As with all creams and oils, if you get any rash or skin reactions when using them, discontinue their use.

Chapter Summary

To do the **first facial cleaning method**, you need the following creams.

- Salicylic Acid
- Glycolic Acid
- Benzoyl peroxide
- Moisturizer

- Night Cream

Before you start using Salicylic acid, you need to do an herbal or water face steaming.

Each of these creams needs to be applied in a certain way.

With the **salicylic acid,** you want to use it in the morning and evening.
The **glycolic acid** is used only in the morning.

The **benzoyl peroxide** is used only in the evening.

In the evening after using benzoyl peroxide, use a **moisturizing cream**, just before you go to bed.

After you have gotten rid of your acne, you can use glycolic acid for a few weeks after to help stabilize your skin.

Use a moisturizing acne cream like **Scotty's Acne Cream,** to help you keep your face clear of acne and to maintain a smooth skin. Adding tree tea oil or Krill oil to this cream will help to maintain a balance of good and bad bacteria in your follicles.

Chapter 23: Second Acne Facial Method

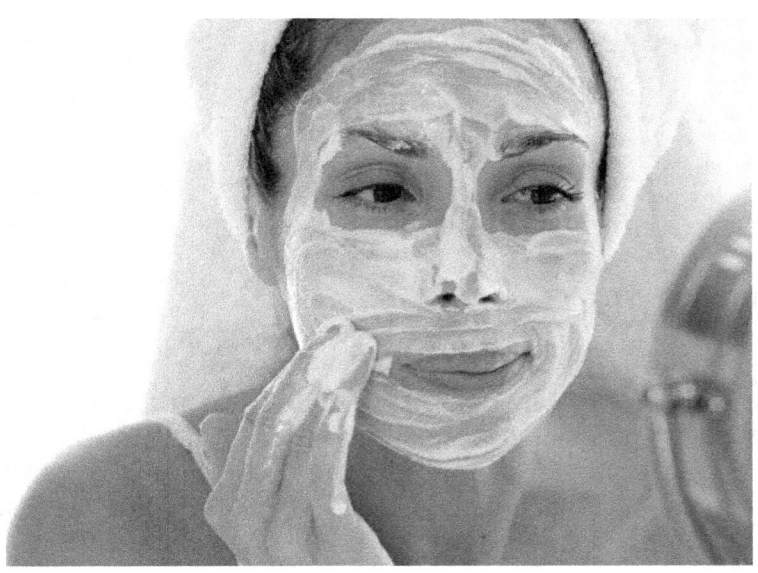

Natural Facial Cleansing

Here is what you will need for this facial. You want to do this for six weeks. Get to enjoy and look forward to doing these facials, since they are quite beneficial for your skin. They will give your skin a chance to recover from bacteria, dirt, and inflammation.

Here is what you will need for this facial.

1. Glycerin soap
2. Herbs: oregano, ginger, and caffeine-free green tea bag
3. Lemon
4. Sea salt
5. Baking soda, Baking Powder

6. Aloe Vera Gel

7. Bentonite clay mask

8. Facial steamer or pot for herbal steam

9. Towel

10. Vitamin E

11. Scotty's or Rich's MSM Lotion

Starting Your Facial Cleansing

Preparing Your Mixtures

Prepare Bentonite clay by adding apple cider vinegar to it. In 1/2 cup, add two tablespoons of cider and mix. You will use this mixture all week or longer.

Mix together a teaspoon of sea salt, five tablespoons of baking soda, and one tablespoon of baking powder. This is a facial scrub.

Herbal Steaming

This herbal steaming is to done for 2 days on and 2 days off. On the off days you will use facial steaming, which does not use herbs, but uses just plain boiling water. This give you face a rest from the herbs and make the herbs more effective the next time you use them.

The first step is to start boiling 5 cups or more of water. Put green tea, plenty of pieces of ginger, and a heaping tablespoon of oregano leaf into the boiling pot of water.

Let the water and herbs boil for about 10 minutes.

As soon as the herbs are ready, wash your face with glycerin soap.

Place the hot pot with herbs on a surface that will not burn or spot. Place a towel over your head and move over the hot herb pot to steam your face.

Caution: Keep a safe distance away from the hot pot and steam, so that you don't burn your
skin. Your skin will start to sweat as your pores open.

Breathe in deeply with your nose and exhale through your mouth, so that the steam can get into your lungs to get the herbal steam benefit.

Steam your face with these herbs for 4-5 minutes.

When you are finished steaming, take a cup and fill it with 1/2 hot tea and 1/2 water, to make it warm. Rinse your face, with this warm tea three times

Pat yourself dry with a towel.

NOTE: You will do this herbal steam cleanse for only two days. Then do two days of facial steaming, with just boiling water.

Water Facial Steaming

After two days of using the herbal steaming, you will do a plain water steam, without herbs, for two days. So, you will be alternating with 2 days herbal steam and 2 day plain water steam. After 2 days of water steam, go back to the herbal steaming.

You are now ready to start the Bentonite clay facial treatment. Bentonite Clay Mask

Take the prepared **Calcium Bentonite clay** and gently rub it all of your face.

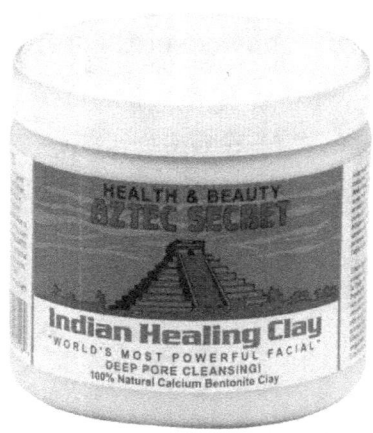

Close your eyes and rub it around your eyes.

Just put on a thin layer. Leave this mask on, for 15 to 20 minutes.

After 20 minutes, wash your face with Glycerin soap and water. When you have cleaned off the Bentonite, rinse your face off with a cup of warm herbal water. Use the hot herbal tea that is leftover from your facial steaming. If you were doing the water facial steaming, rinse your face off with warm water. Then, wash your face with glycerin soap.

Baking Soda Scrub

Pat your face dry and now put the baking soda and salt scrub on your face. Use short circular motions with your fingers. Put a slight pressure on your fingers, so that you give your face a slight scrub. Leave this scrub on your face, for 1 to 2 minutes. Then wash your face with Glycerin soap. Now, again do a final rinse with the herbal tea or water.

Lemon Juice Aloe Vera Application

Squeeze some lemon juice on your hand, and then place it all over your face. Then, let it dry without a towel.

After the lemon has dried, 2–3 minutes, spread 98% pure aloe vera on your face. If you have an aloe vera plant, break off a small section, open the section up and rub the open section all over your face.

Once the aloe vera has dried, you can open up a **capsule of vitamin E.** Place the vitamin E on your fingers and rub it all over your face.

Night Moisturizer

If you don't have vitamin E, you can use a night moisturizer, like Scotty's acne cream or
Rich's MSM lotion. Now, you are ready to go to bed.

Make sure you use a sun screen product, when you go out during the day. You can put Scotty's cream first and then put your sun screen.

This facial cleanse will take about an hour, so set aside this time before bed time.

If you have a partner doing this cleanse with you, they can help you keep on track. If not, keep yourself motivated, and you will see changes at the end of each week that you do the facial cleanse.

Chapter Summary

This cleanse is a great cleanser for the skin. The steps start with washing your face with glycerin soap.

Then, using an herbal green tea, ginger, and oregano, you will do a facial steam for 4 to 5 minutes. This will be followed by a Bentonite clay mask. Then you will do a facial scrub.

Use the herbal tea or water to rinse off your face. As a final step, use lemon, aloe vera and vitamin E or a night cleansing cream or lotion, just before you go to bed.

Rotate your facial steaming every two days, between the herbal and hot water steam.

Chapter 24: Third Acne Facial Cleansing

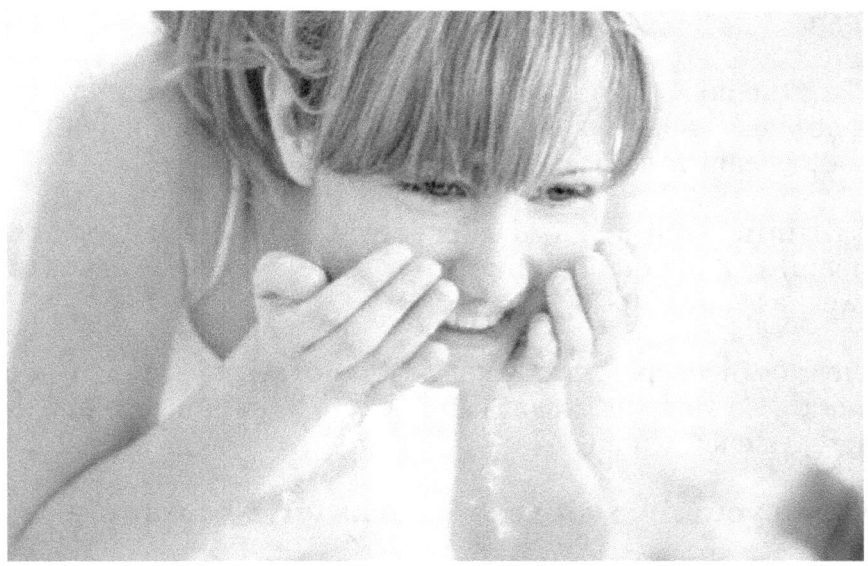

This is What You Need

1. Herbs: oregano, ginger, and caffeine-free green tea bag
2. Pot to steam herbs or facial steamer, Towel

Buy some Bragg's Apple Cider Vinegar
Buy a complexion brush or some large soft cotton balls (or you can use your clean finger tips)

Jojoba oil with 10% or so of tree tea oil, or one bottle of each oil and mix them.

Herbal Steaming

The first step is to start boiling 5 cups or more of water. Put green tea, plenty of pieces of ginger, and a heaping tablespoon of oregano leaf into a boiling pot of water.

Let water and herbs boil about 10 minutes.

As soon as the herbs are ready, wash your face with glycerin soap.

Place the hot pot with herbs on a surface that will not burn or spot. Place a towel over your head and move over the hot herb pot to steam your face.

Caution: Keep a safe distance away from the hot pot and steam, so that you don't burn your skin. Your skin will start to sweat as your pores open.

Breathe in deeply with your nose and exhale through your mouth, so that the steam can get into your lungs to get the herbal steam benefit.

Steam your face with these herbs for 4-5 minutes.

Now, take a cup and fill it with 1/2 hot tea and 1/2 water, to make it warm. Rinse your face with this warm tea three times Pat yourself dry with a towel.

You are now ready to start the Apple Cider facial treatment.

Mixing the Apple Cider Vinegar

Use this facial, when called for in the step by step program.

Once you pat your face dry, you can start using apple cider vinegar either full strength or 1/3 distilled water and 2/3 apple cider vinegar. You can choose the strength that you like. Test your reaction to full strength in a small area of your face and gradually work up to a larger area. If you show no skin allergies or reactions, use the full strength of apple cider vinegar.

Using Apple Cider Vinegar

Now, pour full-strength apple cider vinegar mixture onto your fingers, and massage it onto your face for a few minutes, to check your sensitivities.

Now, dip the complexion brush, cotton pads, or clean fingers into the apple cider vinegar mixture and softly scrub your face to remove dirt and dead skin.

Caution: The cotton pads will absorb a lot of liquid, so you want to carefully not to drip all over your face or counter. You may want to experiment with a facial sponge or another type of soft material.

It may be easier for you to dip your fingers in the cider mixture and then rub it on your face. Just make sure you clean your hands with glycerin soap.

Caution: When scrubbing your face with this mixture be careful not to get it into your eyes. If you need to scrub your forehead, lean your head and down. Use a cotton ball that is not dripping, since the mixture will drip all over your face. Just go slow, until you see how to us this mixture.

If you get it into your eyes, flush them out, with water right away.

The apple cider vinegar will leave your skin slightly acidic, and this is the normal pH balance for your skin. An acid skin will prevent bacteria and other pathogens from getting past your skin barrier. An alkaline skin will breed bacteria.

Do this skin cleansing, with the apple cider vinegar, morning and evening.

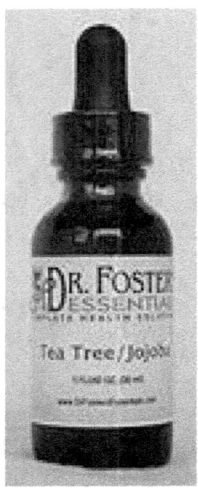

After using the apple cider vinegar, rinse your face a few times with the herbal tea, you used for the herbal steaming. Then pat your face dry. Make sure your towel does not have a lot of detergent or softener reside.

Let your face dry for 5 minutes or so, after your cider vinegar application and rinse. Use 10 drops of jojoba oil to one or two drops of tree tea oil on your hands. Spread this mixture all over your face. Or, you can get **Dr. Foster's blend**s of jojoba-tree tea oil.

The nice thing about jojoba oil is that its composition is close to your sebum oil that comes out of our pores. When you use jojoba, your follicles think your skin is moisturized, so it does not release more sebum oil.

Now, tree tea oil will help smooth out your skin and help to reduce the appearance acne scars. But, always dilute tree tea oil with another oil to prevent it burning your skin. In addition, tree tea oil is known to contain chemicals similar to female sex hormones, which interfere with male and female hormones.

Alert: Young boys and girls should avoid tree tea oil in any type of cosmetic product.

You can go to your health store and buy a bottle jojoba and a bottle of tree tea oil. Mix these two, by adding 2 parts of tree tea to 10 parts jojoba oil.

You can also use coconut oil, instead of jojoba. Use the pure refined coconut oil.

If you have bought Scotty's acne cream or MSM lotion you can use this cream in place of jojoba oil.

You can buy a clean brown dropper bottle at the health-food store, so you can combine the jojoba and tree tea oil.

With a cue tip or cotton ball, softly apply the jojoba oil mixture to your acne area.

Leave this on during the day.

Chapter Summary

In this cleanse you will be using an herbal steam facial and **Bragg's apple cider vinegar**, a soft cotton bud or cotton balls, and jojoba oil mixed with tree oil.

This is an easy cleanse, and you should do it in the morning and in the evening, when called for in the program steps.

Once you cleanse your face with cider, dry it and put **jojoba oil** on your face.

Young boys or girls should avoid using tree tea oil, because of its interference with female and male hormones.

Chapter 25: Alkaline Diet That Helps Stop Acne

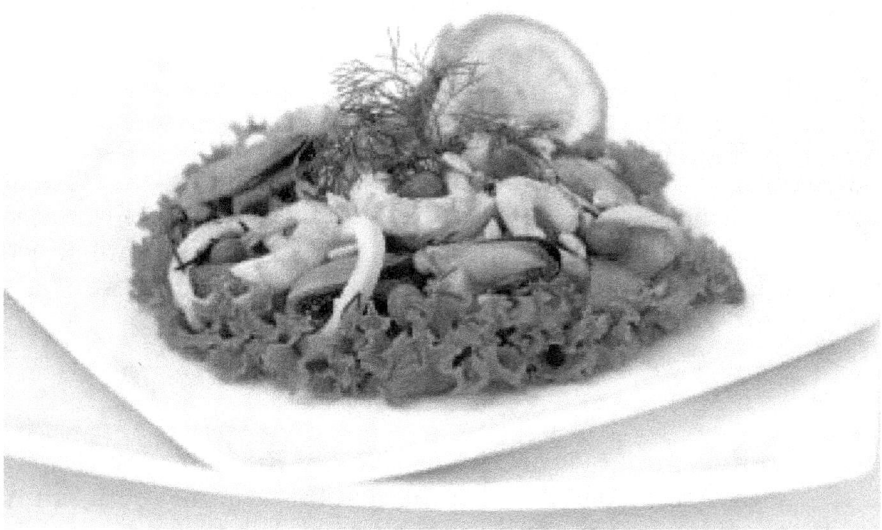

An Acid Body

If you have an acid body, it will take time to make your body alkaline. There are many things you need to change, to have an alkaline body. You need to,

- Eat more alkalizing food

- Eat less acid food

- Neutralize existing body acid and waste

- Neutralize daily acids that enter the body

- Neutralize acids produced by cell metabolism

- Neutralize acids created by body exercise

- Neutralize acids created by negative thinking

- Neutralize acids created by illness

Moving your body more toward alkalinity is what will help you keep acne away. If you have an acid body, it will be hard to maintain healthy skin. An acid body attracts diseases and pathogens, which produces toxins that are acidic.

Mineral Food

The minerals you need to make your body alkaline are sodium, potassium, calcium, phosphorus, and magnesium. These minerals bind with acid, so that they can be eliminated through your elimination channels. All of these minerals need to come from food and supplements. These minerals are called **acid binding minerals**.

Acid Binding

Acid binding minerals are found mostly in high quantitiesin fruits and vegetables. These minerals are sodium, potassium, calcium, magnesium, and phosphorus. What acid binding means is when you eat fruits with these minerals, they will combine with acids in your body and neutralize them. These neutralized acids will be then be eliminated from your body, in your urine and feces.

So you can see the importance of getting a lot of acid binding minerals into your body. Without them, acids would not get eliminated, from your body. They would remain in your body tissues and continue their bodily damage.

Alkaline Binding

Now, there is another side to this story. You have acid binding, and you have alkaline binding. There are minerals that become alkaline binding. These minerals are sulphur, iodine, phosphorus, bromine, fluorine, copper, and silicon. These minerals when digested by a cell will produce a salt that will bind with acid binding minerals (the alkalizing minerals) and eliminate them from your body.

When alkaline minerals are trapped by an acid salt, the alkaline mineral is removed from your body, and your body becomes more acidic. This is the condition you are trying to avoid.

Foods that are alkaline binding and remove the minerals that you need to make your body alkaline are meat, carbohydrates, junk food, all food in packages and cans and some vegetables and some fruits.

Acid Thoughts

Now, we have talked about acid toxins in your body that are brought in through food and the environment. But there is another factor that creates acid in your body, and that is emotions that are activated through life stresses, work pressures, divorce, friendship problems, martial issues, and other similar situations.

These emotional problems create acidic molecules that embed themselves into your tissues just like food acids. These acid molecules can be neutralized with minerals.

Acid Binding Foods

Here is a list of the fruits that have the highest acid binding minerals and the ones that you should be eating to eliminate your body's acids.

The percentage assigned to these fruits is based on fresh fruits that are organic, and that they are not cooked, canned or mixed with sugar.

Fruits above 50% in value are more acid binding, which means they will trap acid wastes better. You will want to eat and drink more of those fruits that are above 51%.

The fruits that are at 50% at are neutral. They are not acid binding nor alkaline binding.

Here is the list of fruits to eat and drink in the order of priority.

Fruits that Bind Acid

1. **Fruits at 100% Acid Binding – Best fruits To Eat**
   Lemons, melons – any type, watermelon

2. **Fruits at 93% Acid Binding – great fruits To Eat**
   Cantaloupes, dried dates, dried figs, limes, mango, papaya

3. **Fruits at 87% Acid Binding – still Great Fruits To Eat**
   Kiwis, passion fruit, pineapples, raisins, umeboshi plums

4. **Fruits at 80% Acid Binding – eat These Fruits**
   Apricots, avocados, bananas, fresh dates, fresh figs, currants, gooseberries, grapes, grapefruits, guavas, kumquats, nectarines, pears, persimmons, quince, berries, cactus

5. **Fruits at 73% Acid Binding – still Fruits To Eat**
   Apples, oranges, peaches, pomegranate, raspberries, sour grapes, strawberries, carob

6. **Fruits at 67% Acid Binding – still Neutralizes Acids**
   Cherries, fresh coconut

Other Food that is Acid Binding

Herbal Teas From Leaves at 73% to 86% acid binding
Alfalfa, mint, sage, spearmint, raspberry strawberry comfrey
7. **All Herbs and Spices at 67% to 73% Acid Binding**

Fruits At 40% to 47% Alkaline Binding - eat less of these fruits Blueberries, cranberries, plums, prunes

Vegetables that Bind Acids

Here is the list of vegetables to eat in order of priority. All of these vegetables will neutralize acid, since they contain minerals that are acid binding.

8. **Vegetables at 93% Acid Binding – best vegetables to eat**
   Kelp, Seaweed, Watercress, Asparagus

9. **Vegetables at 80% Acid Binding – still the best to eat**
   Lettuce Leaf, Oyster plant, Pumpkin, Spinach, Squash, Peas, Carrots, Celery, Chard, Swiss, Dandelion greens

10. **Vegetables at 73% Acid Binding – great vegetables to eat**
    Bamboo shoots, Beets, Broccoli, Cabbage, Cauliflower, Collards, Corn, sweet, Ginger (fresh), Mushrooms, Mustard greens, Onions, Pepper, Potatoes, Green, Lima, String, Potatoes

11. **Vegetables at 67% Acid Binding – eat plenty of these**
    Brussel sprouts, Cucumbers, Eggplants, Okra, Onions, Radishes, Tomatoes

12. **Vegetable juices at 80% to 93% Acid Binding**
    Parsley, wheat grass, carrot, celery, etc.

13. **Soy Bean Products at 60% Acid Binding – limit your use of tofu since it is a genetically modified organism, GMO**

Dried beans, Soy cheese, Soy milk, Tempeh, Tofu
Misc. Acid Binding Food

14. Starches at 80% Acid Binding

Arrowroot flour

15. Sugar at 73% acid Binding
Honey

16. Nuts and Seeds at 60 % to 67% Acid Binding
Almonds, sesame seeds, Granola, Essene Bread, Chestnuts

17. Misc. foods at 60% Acid Binding
Horseradish, Amaranth, Millet, Quinoa, Dried beans, Soy cheese, Soy milk,

NOTE: The lower the alkaline binding percentage, the more that food produces acid in your body.

18. All oils are basically at 50% and are considered neutral.
This includes almond, avocado, canola, coconut, corn castor, olive, soy, sunflower oil.

19. Beans, starches, and nuts and seeds are at 40% to 46% Alkaline Binding
Aduki, Black, Broadbean, Garbanzo, Mung, Pinto, Barley, Corn Meal, Lentils, Brans, Cashews, Coconut (dried), Pecans, Brans, Millet, Filberts, Walnuts, Pumpkin, Sunflower

20. Starches are at 26 to 33 % Alkaline Binding
Brown Rice, Buckwheat, Oats, Spelt, Wheat Whole, Peanuts, corn, rye

21. Rice at 20% Alkaline Binding
White rice

22.   Sugar at 13% Alkaline Binding
White beet or cane sugar

Meat and Fish that Are Alkaline binding
23.   Meat at 26% alkaline binding
Fish With fins and scales, Shellfish - shrimp, scallops, crab lobster, oyster

24.   Meat at 20% Alkaline Binding
Chicken, turkey, rabbit

25. Meat at 13% Alkaline Binding
Beef, goat, pork, lamb

26. All oils are basically at 50% and are considered neutral.
This includes almond, avocado, canola, coconut, corn castor, olive, soy, sunflower oil

27. Misc. Products at 13% to 26% Alkaline Binding
Liquor, wine, beer, coffee, black tea, caffeine drinks

You should be eating 80% acid binding foods and 20% alkaline binding foods. When you eat with this 80/20 formula, you will have an alkaline body, over a period of time. Just gradually work toward this formula.

These are the basic eating principle you should use to achieve ultimate health. In the next chapter, you will get information how to eat.

Chapter Summary

An **acid body favors parasites**, diseases, and acne. To get rid of acne, you will need to move your acid body into a more alkaline condition. If you have acne and an acid body, it will be difficult for you to eliminate your acne, until you create an alkaline body.

An acid body holds acid waste and toxins in lymph, tissue, muscles, and cells. This acid waste needs to be neutralized and eliminated from your body.

Eating acid binding food or minerals or less acid food, will help you change our body, to a more alkaline condition.

To **neutralize body acids**, you need to eat fruits and vegetables that are packed with sodium potassium, calcium, phosphorus and magnesium.

The **best alkalizing foods are** lemons, melons, watermelon, cantaloupes, figs, mangos and papaya. In vegetables, the best alkalizing foods are kelp, seaweed, watercress, asparagus, pumpkin, spinach squash, carrots, celery, and dandelion.

A list of **acid foods** is provided in this chapter.

To achieve an alkaline body, move your eating pattern to 80% alkaline food to 20% acid food.

Chapter 26: Breakfast That Keeps You Acne Free - Cycle 1

Natural Body Cycles

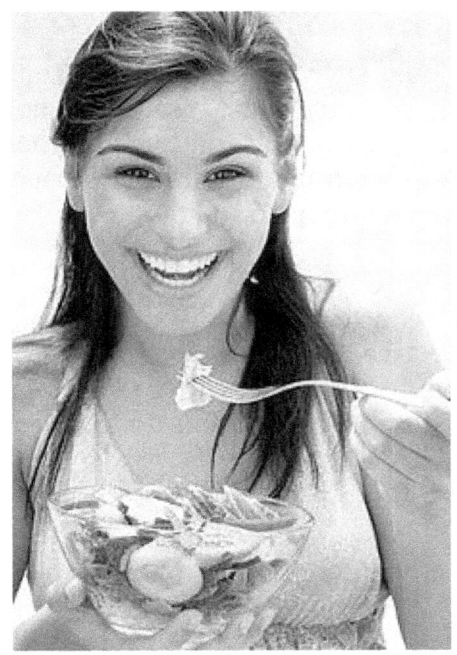

Your body has three cycles. It has an internal body regeneration and toxic removal time or cycle. Then, it has a time where it wants to eliminate the accumulated toxic matter from your body. And, finally, it has a time that it needs to intake food for cycle regeneration and daily functioning.

First Body Cycle 6 am to Noon

Your first body cycle occurs from 6 am to noon. This is called the elimination–detoxification cycle. It is a time where your body removes body wastes that have accumulated during your third body cycle. To help the first body cycle, you need to eat foods that are digested quickly and that do not block your elimination channels.

The acid and toxic wastes your body has gathered during the night need to be eliminated, when you wake. This is done by urinating, bowel movements, sweating, and hard breathing. Keeping the nightly toxins in your body, leads to the creation of more toxins, acid accumulation, body stress, and illness.

Blocking Your First Body Cycle

Each day, you have a chance to detoxify your body from 6 am to noon. You can block this detoxification, if you eat food that takes more than three to four hours to digest.

A breakfast made of heavy foods, such as eggs, cereal, toast, sausage, ham, bacon, potatoes, oats, tortillas, biscuits, bagels, donuts, and sweet breads block your elimination channels. Your body is trying to use these channels to eliminate waste, accumulated during the night, and you need to help it.

Helping Your First Body Cycle

In the morning to noon, you need to eat food and drink that moves fast through your digestive tract, and that pulls out toxic matter that is stored in your body. Food that travels fast through your body puts pressure in body areas to push out toxins.

Here's how this is done.

In the morning, you need to drink water, fruit or vegetable juices. You need to drink an herbal tea, chlorophyll drink, green tea, or a green drink. You also need to eat raw fruits and vegetables or slightly cooked vegetables. Eating like this doesn't disrupt your first natural cycle.

Your body wants to urinate and have bowel movements in the morning, but any heavy food you eat in the morning interferes with this process. A heavy breakfast causes your body to concentrate on digesting this food, instead of concentrating on eliminating nightly waste accumulations.

Having liquid, fruits or vegetables for breakfast, helps you promote a bowel movement and to release urine. Also liquids or fruits only take an hour or so to digest, whereas solid food can take up to 3 to 4 hours and by that time you are ready for lunch.

What to Drink in the Morning

Test your urine pH first thing in the morning. Do this for four days and then do another 4 days a month later. You can then see the progress of this diet.

When you get up in the morning, drink any of the following drinks. Vary your drinks after a few days.

- 8 oz. of water from the juice of one lemon

- 8 oz. of water from the juice of one lemon and one lime

- 8 oz. of mixed fresh lemon, orange, and grapefruit

- 8 oz. of water from the juice of one lemon and 1-2 oz. of chlorophyll

- 1 cup of decaffeinated green tea with add slices of ginger

- 1 cup of your favorite green powder

You can use any other health drink you like, as long as it contains water, no sugar, or artificial sweetener. To make some drinks more palatable, you can use a few drops of honey, until you get used to the taste. Use honey only on your green drink or herbal tea.

If you like to make a power smoothie, this is the time to do it. You can check out the smoothies at the end of this book.

After Your Morning Drink

After you finish your morning drink, wait about 1/2 hour before you start your breakfast. Eat only fruits or vegetables, for breakfast.

Use the chart from the **Alkaline Diet chapter 28**, to determine which fruits and vegetables to use. Do not eat raw fruits with raw vegetables.

Mix fruits that are 90% or more acid binding with those that lower acid binding.

You can mix the juices of fruits and vegetables to make the vegetables more palatable.

Here are a few morning breakfast suggestions:

- Cut and prepare a bowl of various fresh fruits. Do not add any toppings or sweeteners.

- Cut and mix watermelon and cantaloupe slices together. Do not mix this fruit with other types of fruit.

- Prepare a "only" vegetable soup with the best acid binding vegetables. Put the extra in a thermos for later. You can prepare this soup the day before.

- Prepare a fruit pudding in a blender using three or four different fruits listed in the Alkaline Diet chapter 28. This will help to quench your hunger. Use different fruits on different days. Put the extra pudding in a thermos for your morning break.

- Prepare a juice mixture of carrots and apples. You can add other vegetables to get a strong and nutritious drink.

- Prepare a smoothie, as shown in the smoothie chapter. Drink part of it for breakfast and use the rest for your breaks.
- Drink a lemon and chlorophyll drink
- Drink a green drink

On occasion, it's ok to eat a heavy breakfast. You can eat eggs, potatoes or a small amount of whole oats, not the quick-cooking oats. You can use apple juice to dilute the oats and add a banana and raisins. Your body can deal with an occasion heavy breakfast.

Fruit Pudding Recipe

Here is a typical fruit pudding recipe you can use. The Smoothie Chapter has more puddings you can make simply by not put in so much liquid.

Eat some of this pudding in the morning or take it to work for your breaks. Here are two different things you can do with a blender.

Put into a blender,

- Two small or one large banana
- One mango
- Pineapple
- One apple
- 1/4 of a papaya (if available)
- Powdered vitamin C from two to three capsules
- A tablespoon of lecithin

- Small amount of apple juice to make this blend into a pudding

Blend all of this for 1 – 2 minutes.
Pineapple Smoothie
Mix the following in a blender to create a smoothie.

- 1-2 cups of fresh pineapples

- 1/2 cups apple slices

- 1/4 cup fresh apple juice

- 1/4 cup rice dream or almond milk (as needed)

- 1 small banana

- 1-teaspoon lecithin

- 1-teaspoon flax seed oil

- 2 teaspoons bran (oat or rice)

- Full cup of plain yogurt

Morning Snack time

During your morning and afternoon breaks, it's time to open your thermos and have a good snack. Make sure you take your snack breaks. Use only fruits, vegetables, nuts, and soups for your snacks. These types of snacks help you to digest your food better and also activate peristaltic colon action. They give you fiber and many of the minerals you need, to make your body more alkaline.

Use drinks like apple, cherry, prune, pineapple, tomato, carrot, and so on, to improve your regularity.

There you have it, the breakfast. Start using this breakfast method and add your own creations, using fruits and vegetables.

Check Chapter

Chapter Summary

You have **body cycles** where your body is busy doing detoxification - elimination, digestion, and rejuvenation.

The **first cycle is from 6 am to noon** and during this period, your body is detoxifying and eliminating waste from your body.

When you eat a heavy meal, you block this elimination time and reduce the bowel movements and urination that you might have. By eating lite foods such as fruits, vegetables and their juices, during the morning, you assist your body during this elimination cycle. Fruits and vegetables and their juices digest fast and move through your body within a few hours.

The **best breakfast** you can have is fruits, special juices, and fruit smoothies. You can also have vegetable juices and certain vegetables.

Use these **easy to prepare fruits recipes** to start your day and to help detoxify your body and assist in your elimination of waste. If you have diabetes or want to back off on sugar, drink more vegetable juices and mix them with apple juice.

Chapter 27: Acne Free With Body Cycles 2 And 3

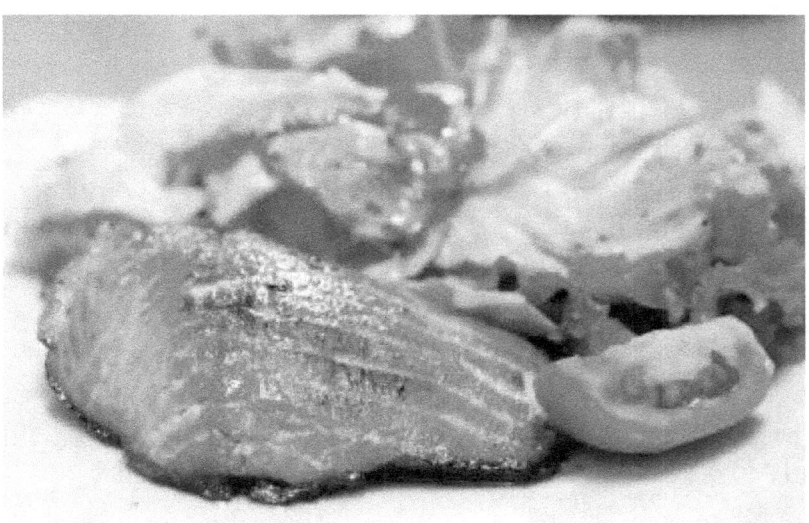

Second Body Cycle Noon to 8 pm

The second body cycle is the eating and digestion cycle. This cycle is from noon to 8 pm and is the time for you to eat nutritious food. Choosing the food for your meals is critical, because this will determine the level of health that you have or will have. When you eat the wrong kind of food, expect to be sick.

Now that you have eliminated waste, during your morning elimination and detoxification time, it is time to have a good lunch and dinner.

Cycle 2 is the time when your body should be taking in food and digesting. During this period, is time to eat solid food. What you eat has to be in alignment with what your stomach can do. Your stomach can only work on one solid food or protein at a time, so your lunch and dinner should only have one solid food. A lunch can consist of,

- chicken and a green salad

- fish or tuna and a green salad

- shrimp and a green salad

- beef and a green salad

- protein and a green salad

Every heavy meal you eat should always have some raw vegetables or slightly cooked ones to complement your main course. Various sauces can be added to your meal.

If you eat meat or carbohydrate such as rice, potatoes, noodles, these foods do not have
fiber. You need fiber to help process and digest these foods. So that, during the night cleansing cycle, the undigested food will be ready to come out the next day.

Eating for Cycle 2

Any eating habit that disrupts cycle 2, the eating and digestion cycle, affects the other cycles. Here's how you can help your body's cycle 2 to be more effective. Eat in this manner for lunch and dinner.

- Eat only one solid food with vegetables during lunch or dinner. Lunch can be one meat or seafood with a fresh vegetable salad. It can be one carbohydrate with sauce and salad with dressing.

- Limit the amount of water you drink during your eating. Excess water will dilute your digestive acids and slow down digestion of your food. It may even cause you to have incomplete digestion of protein.

- Eliminate drinking any sodas, coffee, tea or water, during your meals. If you need to clear your dry throat, use a bit of room-temperature water.

- Eating meals with more than one solid food, such as meat and potatoes, chicken and rice, fish and rice, chicken and noodles, eggs and toast, cheese and bread will diminish the energy, you need during cycle 1, the elimination cycle.

- It is permissible to eat beef and chicken at the same time, but not chicken and eggs or beef and nuts or chicken and beans. Eat the same type of protein at the same time, but do not mix different proteins.

It's ok to eat different types of carbohydrates at the same time, with a salad, but not with protein, since carbohydrates digest easier and faster than protein.

Eating as outline above is a new way of thinking, about how to eat. In the beginning, it will be hard for you not eat beef, without carbohydrates. But, you should consider eating fewer carbohydrates, with your meat, as time passes.

Eating the right combination of foods at mealtime helps to preserve your energy for the elimination cycle and prevents you from creating spoiled food, in your stomach, that is converted to acid waste. It is this acid waste that results in illness and fat. This is the reason most people, as they age, become fat or come down with various illnesses that terminate their lives early.

Lunch time

For lunch, you want to make sure you have a salad that has the vegetables listed in the Alkaline Diet Chapter. And, make sure you include the dark-green lettuce, tomato, cucumber, and celery.

Meat to Eat

You can chose any meat that you want, such as ground lean meat, filet mignon, T-bone, sirloin, tenderloin, lamb, veal. But, don't over load on the meat. You only need a couple of ounces, unless you do physical work. If you like fish, this is the best protein you can eat. Fish protein takes longer to digest, so it is better to eat it for lunch instead of for dinner. Try to eat fish, at least two times a week.
Here is a list of meats you can eat. Use 2 to 3 oz. of meat.

- Poultry: chicken or turkey (white or dark meat, No skin), Cornish hen, no skin

- Fish: fresh or frozen cod, flounder, haddock, Halibut, trout, lox, tuna fish (fresh or canned in water)

- Shellfish: clams, crab, lobster, scallops, shrimp

- Beef: USDA select or choice grades of lean beef trimmed of fat, such as round, sirloin, flank steak, tenderloin, roast (rib, chuck, rump), steak (T-bone, porterhouse, cubed)

- Lamb: roast chop or leg

- Veal: Lean chop, roast

- Salmon (fresh or canned)

- Sardines (canned)

- Tuna (canned in oil, drained)

Brown Rice and Meat

For lunch, you can eat a small amount of brown rice and 4 oz. of meat. This meat can be beef, lamb, veal, chicken, turkey, or fish. Do not fry any of this meat. It is best to bake or broil this meat. Try to eat more fish or sea food than any of the other types of meat. Use a small amount of rice. But, it is best to eat meat with salad, since this will give you the best digestion.

You can also eat cottage cheese, with fresh fruit.

Dinner Time

For dinner, you can have meat and salad. It is best to have the same type of protein you had for lunch. This will help you digest your food better. So, if you have chicken for lunch, have chicken for dinner.

You don't even have to have any meat, or have very little, for dinner. You can have rice, soup, and salad. Or you can have a cup full of rice and a pouched egg. You can also add some chili sauce into a pan and break an egg into the sauce after it is hot and cook the egg and add it to your brown rice.

If you don't want to have a salad, then cook some vegetables, from the acid binding vegetable list. Use a little water and cook the vegetables just long enough, to get them slightly soft.

Use beans to make a bean fresh salad.

Fatty Foods

Here is a list of fat you can eat. For a healthy diet, you need to eat some fat both saturated and unsaturated. But, you have to go easy on eating saturated fat and not go overboard.

Saturated Fat

- Butter, stick
- Butter, reduced-fat
- Coconut, sweetened, shredded

- Coconut milk
- Cream cheese: Regular or Reduced-fat
- Sour cream:
- Avocado, medium
- Nuts: almonds, cashews, mixed (50%peanuts)
- hazelnut
- Pecans
- walnuts, pecans, Brazil nuts
- Peanut butter, smooth or crunchy without sugar
- Sesame seeds
- Pumpkin or sunflower seeds

Drinking Water, Juices, and Eating Fruits
Do not eat fruits immediately after your meals. Eat them about one hour after. Fruits and juices should be used as between meal snacks or for breakfast.

Drink as least 6 cups of distilled water or ROI water every day. Since you are eating fruits and juices, you are getting plenty more water.

Afternoon Snack Time

If you have any leftover protein from lunch, use them as a snack. You can also eat fruit or juices that will help make you alkaline. By eating these types of snacks, you will be less hungry, during lunch or dinner.

When Hungry

For breaks, eat fruits and juices that give you alkaline minerals. But, don't eat fruits and juices with your meals, unless they are vegetable juices. Don't drink large quantities of juices, since they are high in fructose, which is converted to excess fat during your digestion. Do drinking and eating in moderation.

Near Bed Time

Don't eat two to three hours before bed time. If you get hungry during this time, drink some juice or have a small portion of fruit such as pineapple or any other fruit.

Desserts You Can Eat

These are the low-carbohydrate desserts you can eat.

FRUITS

- Jell-O or Agar Agar (add banana, berries, cantaloupe, peaches, or pineapple to the Jell-O) no sugar, but you can add a touch of honey
- Banana Custer without sugar
- Banana with skimmed milk
- Berries with milk
- Apples raw, baked or stewed with some cinnamon

Here is a salad dressing you can make and use on your salads.

- Apple cider vinegar
- Flax seed oil
- Olive oil
- Lecithin granules

Use two times more flax seed oil as olive oil. Use apple cider vinegar to your taste. Use a teaspoon of lecithin to help you digest and absorb these oils better.

Foods to Avoid

Here are some foods that will compromise your health. Avoid them if possible.

- Ice cream
- Canned fruits with sugar
- Gravies
- Mayonnaise
- Salad dressings
- Baked products such as cakes, pies, cookies, donuts
- Alcoholic drinks
- Sodas and all sugary drinks
- All foods in packages or junk food
- All sugary products or desserts
- Jelly or jam
- Frozen foods

Third Body Cycle 8 pm to 6 am

The last body cycle is from 8 pm to 6 am. Try to keep your dinner meals lighter than your lunch. You don't want your body to be digesting your food, during the night, when it should be cleansing and rejuvenating.

In this cycle, your body is absorbing and using the food you have eaten, during the noon to 8 pm period. This is the time the food you have eaten, during the day, is assimilated, absorbed and distributed throughout your body.

Food that was eaten during body cycle 2, and that was combined and eaten properly will digest within three to four hours. Whereas food not combines properly, a meal consisting of protein and carbohydrates can take up to seven to eight hours to pass through the stomach. During this time, your food will putrefy and ferment and become acidic. Under these conditions, you will not get the most nutrients from that meal.

Eat your last meal by 6-7 pm so that your food digests in your stomach, before going to bed. Three hours later, your food will have moved into your small intestine, where it is ready for assimilation. When you go to bed three hours after your last meal, your body will be
absorbing the food you have eaten for dinner. It will be removing acid waste and toxins and placing them in your bladder, colon or skin for the morning elimination.

Remember, anything you do different than what these cycles call for, will disrupt them and cause them to become extended. When this happens, some of your food turns into acid, and you will not absorb the value of your food. You lose energy and become tired, and over time, you gain weight and create serious illnesses.

By midnight and after, your body is busy cleansing and preparing for elimination and detoxification during your morning cycle. Don't block this process by eating a heavy dinner the day before.

Chapter Summary

Cycle 2 is from noon to 8 pm, and it covers your lunch, snacks and dinner.

This is the time to eat the way your body needs food. **For lunch,** you need to **eat one protein** and salad or slightly cooked vegetables. Your stomach digests food better when it has to deal with one protein and not with a protein and carbohydrate. You can eat chicken with salad, fish with salad, beef with salad, or any protein with salad.

If you want **to eat carbohydrates**, then eat one carbohydrate with salad. Don't mix the carbohydrate with protein in a meal. This way of eating is not typical, and it will be hard to get used to it, but it has great benefits for acne. Just work slowly into changing into this diet.

For dinner eat the same way you ate for lunch. Do not mix protein with carbohydrates in your meals. At the same time, don't drink water with your meal.

Cycle 3 is from 8 pm to 6 am. It is this time to prepare for bed and not eat anything. During sleep, body is digesting and absorbing, and cleansing and rejuvenating.

A list of meats and fatty foods you can eat are provided in this chapter.

During your afternoon break, drink or eat fruits. This will help you to digest any remaining food in your stomach and to help you move your food residues into the colon.
Fruits help you to activate peristaltic action and bring about an afternoon bowel movement.

Chapter 28: Sun, Air, and Water for Acne

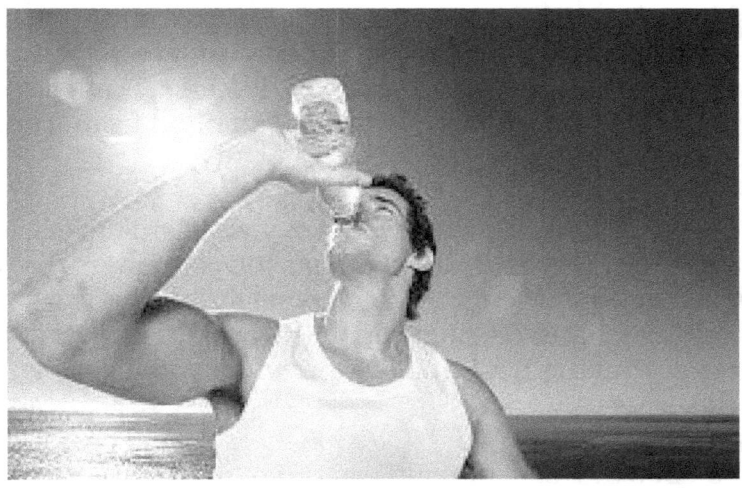

Sun and Air

Expose yourself to plenty of sun and air every day, for about 30 minutes minimum. But, make sure you are using sun screen when you do. Use a hat to prevent your face from being directly in the sun. Go outside every day, if you can, to get plenty of sun and air.

Sun

The sun provides you with plenty of vitamin D3 that you need for good skin. During the winter, it may be hard to get sun, so supplementing with Vitamin D3 is important. In the supplement chapter, you will get the dose for vitamin D3. Vitamin D3 is a major element in the absorption of calcium in your body. Calcium is needed in large quantities to maintain good body function.

Drink More Water

Water provides the basis for all liquids in your body. It also breaks down into oxygen and hydrogen, as your body needs them.

The skin stores around 12% water. It is important to maintain this amount with the correct amount of good fat. Drink around 2 quarts of distilled and or Reverse Osmosis water every day. This can come from plain water and from fruits and vegetables.

Try to use glass containers when buying distilled or reverse osmosis water. Try to avoid using plastic containers for water. These plastic containers contain chemicals left in the container walls during manufacturing, which leaches out into the water. If you are drinking fresh juices, you will also be getting water from these juices.

If you dislike the taste of plain water, you can squeeze the juice from one lemon or any other fruit into your water to give it more flavor.

Air

Air contains 16% oxygen, which helps to keep bacteria and parasites in control. Air pollution is a big problem in many cities, which reduces the oxygen in air and floods toxic particles into your body. So, you want to make sure you are getting a lot of oxygen into your body, from the air you breathe. There are other ways to get oxygen into your body, if you need to.

In your home, you can add filters that eliminate air pollution. You can also buy air ozonators to kill air pathogens and pollution.

Oxygen

All foods contain oxygen. But there are some foods that are higher in oxygen content than others. Foods that have iron in them attract oxygen and have more oxygen. Foods that are high in calcium, potassium, iodine and fluorine also attract oxygen. A diet high in protein, carbohydrates, and fats reduces body oxidation and will harm your body.

Here is the list of foods high in oxygen. Make sure you include these foods in your diet.

- Nuts, seeds, Raisins, Figs

- Beets, Parsnips, Spinach, Carrots, Tomatoes

- Blueberries, Cherry Juice, Grapes

- Green Peppers, Onions, garlic

- Fish

Oxygen is a powerful source throughout your body in that it provides the oxidation needed in tissue and cells. This oxidation is the digestion of nutrients in a cell that provide the cell with energy. As oxygen reduces or metabolizes nutrients and cell waste, it creates free radicals. For this reason, you need fruits, vegetables, and supplements to provide antioxidants that neutralize these free radicals.

One of the most potent free radical eliminators is the antioxidant glutathione, which is created right in your cells. In your cells, glutathione helps to eliminate the free radicals that oxygen creates and that enter the cells from the lymph liquid.

When you are low in glutathione, your immune system is impacted and reduces your ability to control and eliminate acne.

Oxygen gives you life. It enhances metabolism, elevates mind power, improves cell regeneration, and gives you maximum health. It helps your digestion, improves nutrient adsorption, gives you optimism and enthusiasm, and promotes youthful appearance and activity.

Excess oxygen in your body expands most of your physicals and mental abilities. It heightens your emotions, so that you feel angry and happiness at an intense level.

When you have a deficiency of oxygen, you become irritable, stubborn and hypersensitive. You become more susceptible to germ and pathogenic diseases. Your brain becomes dull and you have more congestion, bleeding, stomach problems, and have difficulty breathing.

Chapter Summary

Your skin needs clean sun, air and water. Do not allow the sun to dehydrate your skin, so only remain under the sun for about 20 to 30 minutes per day. Make sure you use sun screen, during the time, you are doing this acne program.

The sun provides the energy to create **vitamin D3** on your skin and then routes it to your small intestine. There it is used to transport calcium into your blood stream. **You need a lot of vitamin D3, 8000 to 10000 IU**. You will not get this with only 20 minutes out in the sun, so take a vitamin D3 supplement.

Drink plenty of water. Water keeps your skin hydrated and keeps you from becoming constipated. Your kidney uses this water to constantly clean your blood, create urine, and maintain your blood's and body's pH.

You need clean air. Contaminated air is trouble for you. Polluted air lacks oxygen, and oxygen kills pathogens and helps your cells digest nutrients for energy.

Eat those foods that are high in oxygen to get more

oxygen into your body. See the list in this chapter.

Chapter 29: Brushing And Keeping Your Skin Clean

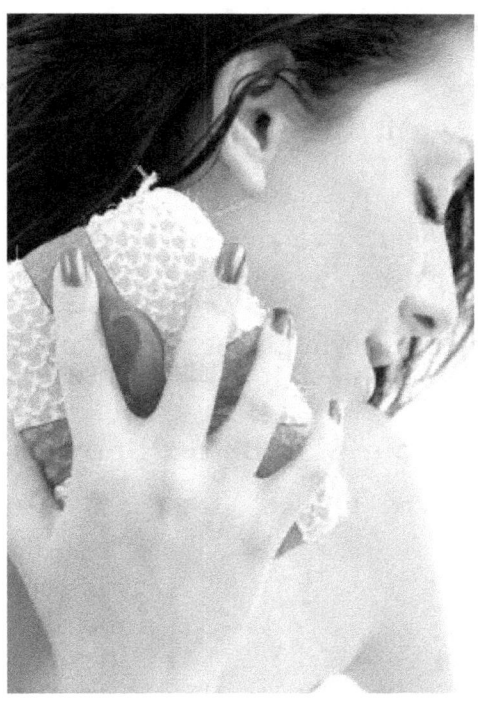

Skin Brushing

Brushing your body skin, before taking a shower, is a way to stimulate your lymphatic system and increase blood circulation. You can brush your skin, with special skin brushes or with a cloth.

Do not brush your facial skin. Improving your body skin function, improves your facial skin function.

Brushing your skin also does the following:

- Removes dry dead cells that can clog your skin

- Opens pores, which allow you to excrete more toxins safely

- Activates the nerves near the top of your skin, making your skin work better

- Stimulates the tiny blood vessels near your skin and brings more nutrients and acid neutralizing minerals to your skin

- Improves your overall health, since the skin must eliminate close to 2 pounds of waste through the pores.

If you practice dry brushing your skin, you will see improved beauty and health in your skin.

How To Brush Your Skin Before Showering

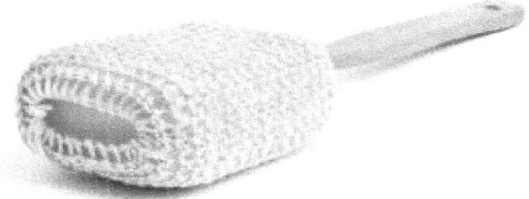 There are two different types of brushes that are designed for dry skin brushing.

- A natural bristle brush
- Loofah with a long handle

Before you take a shower, here's how to dry brush your skin.

Start with a gentle light touch and circular motions at your feet. You should always brush only in the direction of your heart. From the feet upward, brush up towards your heart. At the neck, brush downward towards your heart.

After you finishing brushing, about 5 minutes, take a shower to remove the dead and old skin.

How to Brush Your Skin in the Shower

You can also scrub your skin during your shower. Use a Loofah in the shower with soap and brush your skin as described above. This is a gentler way to brush your skin, and you can wash away the skin derby, at the same time.

When you start bushing for the first time, do it softly and gently, until your skin gets used to the rough feeling.

Because skin brushing promotes the release of toxins through your skin, you want to make sure you are not constipated; otherwise, you will start to release too many toxins through the skin.

A word of caution: Brush only once a day and do not brush too hard. Excessive brushing over stimulates the skin and can produce unwanted side effects.

Keeping Your Face Clean

If you use facial commercial cosmetics, you need to stop. Some cosmetics irritate the skin and can cause acne by plugging up the pores, on your face. This may not happen right away, but over time this will happen. The cosmetic chemicals that can cause you the most irritation and pore inflammation are:

- mineral oil
- lanolin
- parabens
- propylene glycol

Look at the label of the cosmetics you use. You will find that many cosmetics, soaps, and sunscreens contain these chemicals.

You need to get a clean face to start this program. Find a water base make up, not an oil base one that does not irritate your face and use it sparingly.

When you wash your face, don't use any commercial soap, since they are filled with chemicals that will irritate and worsen your condition. And, don't excessive wash your face, as this will dry your skin of the natural protective oils. Also, don't keep touching your face, since you spread or add bacteria to it.

Washing Your Face

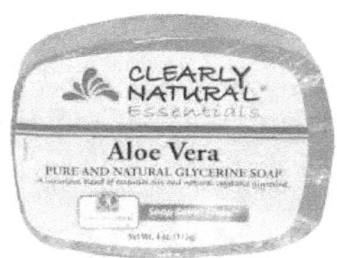

To wash your face, use only Castile hand or liquid soap or Pure **Glycerin hand soap**. You can pat your face with a clean hot face towel to bring circulation, to your face. The hot towel will open your pores and move toxic material out of them.

Then, wash your face with Glycerin soap. Do not scrub hard to burst a pimple.

Use the hot towel application only 2-3 times per week.

When a pimple is open, do not continue to rub or scrub it. In fact, do not pick or scratch an open pimple, since this could create other sores or leave scars that are difficult to remove. Just washing your face with clean soap will keep the surface of your face free of toxic matter.

Keep in mind that whatever you put on your skin, will move into your skin and bloodstream.

During the day or night, avoid resting your cheeks or chin on your hand(s) or arm(s). This can irritate your face and cause acne to breakouts. When you sleep, try to sleep on your back and not with your face or side of your face on or into your pillow.

Herbal Face Wash

After you wash your face with soap, you can use an herbal tea wash, if you like. This is a very simple thing to do and requires only one or two herbs. This herbal tea wash will have a healing and soothing effect on the open acne sores.

Here's what to do

Add one tablespoon of Yarrow Root, slices of ginger and one bag of green tea into a pot with four or more cups of water. Boil the water then let the tea sit 10 -15 minutes off the heater plate. Strain the tea, and after it cools down, you can use it to rinse your face. Do this in the morning, when you first wash your face and just before you go to bed. If you make a big pot of herbal tea, you can save it, for the day's use.

Chapter Summary

Brushing your skin helps to provide blood circulation that brings new nutrients to your follicles. It also helps to remove dirt, cell waste, and bacteria that create skin contamination. It is skin brushing that stimulates your skin to function better.
You can **brush your skin,** before you take a shower or during your shower with a special brush. When you brush your body, always brush with a single stroke towards your heart.

Don't use commercial cosmetic products, because they contain too many chemicals that are bad for your skin and health. Use Glycerin soap, for your face and body. Any product that you put on your skin will find its way into your blood stream.

Herbal face washes are a great way to feed your skin.

Create a tea with the herbs listed and feed your face with minerals, nutrients, anti-oxidants, and anti-bacterial chemicals.

Chapter 30: Twenty Minute Acne Exercise

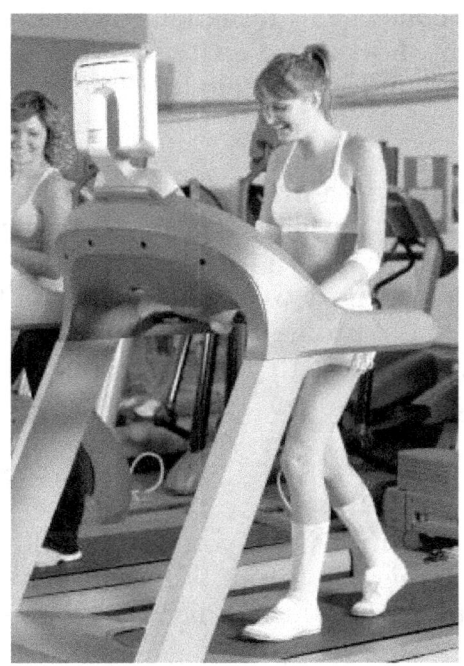

Exercising

So why is it important to do exercise to help eliminate acne?

The main reason is that when you exercise you create more balance in your body, and it starts to give you better health. In addition, you will sweat more, and this helps to eliminate more toxins out of your body. You will strengthen your heart, and it will give you a better life.

Exercise research studies have found that the more physically fit you are the better your body works. The main problem is finding an exercise that you will want to do 3 to 4 times a week and that does not take hours to do.

The Pace Exercise Program

PACE® Exercise Program by Al Sears, MD., is the first and only program conceived, designed, tested and proven to achieve fitness in short timed exercises. It does this, when you do short exercises and build them into longer times and higher intensives.

The key is to start with a brief exertion that is comfortable for you, at your current capacity. It's not so important how hard you exert yourself, when you first start. It's the little bit of exertion that you do next week that you didn't do this week. This is the element of progressivity. By changing your program through time, you work with your metabolism and your ability to force your body to change.

Risk Factors

Here are some conditions that you need to think about, before starting this exercise program. If you have any of these conditions, you may want to discuss exercising with your doctor.

- Over 55 years
- Have asthma or other lung conditions
- Take heart medication
- Have not been exercising for years
- Have any type of heart condition
- Have not seen a doctor for over three years
- Are overweight by 27 pounds or more

When you begin an exercise program, you need to start out slow and each day increase the speed or intensity of your exercise.

Heart Rate Levels

Here is the heart rate chart to use in your exercise. First, compute the minimum and maximum heart rates you should achieve, during or just after you finish exercising. Use the following formula.

- Minimum heart rate = 60% of (220 minus your age.)

- Maximum heart rate = 80% of (220 minus your age.)

Your exercise challenge is to reach the minimum heart rate during your exercise and work up to your maximum heart rate as you exercise harder each day.

Heart Rate Chart

Age	min. HR	max. HR
30	114	152
40	108	144
50	102	136
60	96	128

HR = Heart Rate

Use these heart rates as a guide. Your actual heart rates may be more or less based on your illness, medication, or good health.

If you have a major illness, contact your doctor for exercise information.

The 10-Minute Program

Here's a simple program to use that does not take a lot of time. In this 10-minute program below, you're going to focus on gradually increasing your intensity of exercise each day.

The exercise you will do is based on what you can do at home. If you have a treadmill, then you can do running. If you have an exercise bike, you can do biking. If you have a rebounded, you can do stationary running. If you have no equipment, do jumping jacks. The exercise you do is not the critical thing. The important thing is to get your heart rate up, according to your age.

You are going to do a series of timed exercise. In the formula below, warm up is where you stretch before your exercise. Exercise is the time you do your exercise. Relax is the time where you stop your exercise, so you can recover your heart rate to a normal beat.

(warm up) (exercise) (relax) (exercise) (relax) (exercise) (relax)

Before you start your exercise, measure your heart rate. This is your base rate. Create a log to record it. After your exercise, measure your heart rate again. Use the heart rate chart above to see where you stand with your rate. If your rate is not in the chart, calculate it and record it in your note book. Keeping within your heart rate, indicates you are working your heart in an optimal way.

Week

1 2 min 5 min 3 min   (2 min warm up, 5 min exercise, 3min relax)

2 1 min   3 min 2 min 3 min (1 min warm up, 3 min exercise, 2 min relax, 3 min exercise)

3 1 min   2 min 2 min 2 min 2 min 2 min 2 min

4 1 min   1 min 2 min 1 min 2 min 1 min   2 min

Notice the progression of this workout. Over time, the duration of each exercise period decreases, but you do more intense   exercises. This progression is towards reaching maximal
heart beat for your age. This is the center of the PACE® program.

Here's how it works...

Week One

2 min 5 min 3 min (2 min warm up, 5 min exercise, 3min relax)

During week one, you're going to take it easy and just do one warm-up for 2 minutes and then one exercise set at a low to moderate intensity. Just do what feels comfortable. If you are out of shape, it's okay. You can just start with walking for 5 minutes.   Then relax for three minutes and start walking again.   Do this for 5 sets. But measure and record your heart beat before and after each set.

Try to do this 10-minute interval exercise at least three times during the first week. But, each time you do it, slightly increase the intensity level. By the end of the first week, you should feel like you've given yourself a slight exercise challenge.

Keep in mind that how you adjust the intensity will depend on what instrument you're using.
If you're on a stationary bike, increase the level on the control panel, so it becomes harder to pedal. If you're on an elliptical, boost the incline so it's harder to run, etc.

Week Two

2   1 min 3 min 2 min 3 min (1 min warm up, 3 min

exercise, 2 min   relax, 3 min exercise)

During week two, you'll add another exercise set. But the duration of your exertion periods will decrease. After a quick warm up, you'll do a 3-minute exercise period. As you start, notice how fast you're going, and how long it takes for your heart and lungs to meet the challenge.

When 3 minutes is up, begin your recovery. If you need to stop, that's okay. Otherwise, your recovery period should be a slow, easy pace. If you're on an elliptical machine, for example, you should slow down so you feel like you're walking.

During each recovery period, you should focus on your heart rate, so if you start to pant, it is okay. Feel your lungs quickly fill up and release. Allow your body to come back to a state of rest. This is strengthening your heart and lungs. Measure your heart rate, immediately after your exercise time.

Week Three

3   1 min 2 min 2 min 2 min 2 min 2 min 2 min

During week 3, you'll start with a quick warm up and then a 2-minute exercise period. But, this time, increase the intensity to give yourself more of a challenge.

When 2 minutes is up, begin your recovery. Repeat this exercise process 2 more times. During week 3, try to repeat this workout three or four times.

Week Four

4   1 min 1 min 2 min 1 min 2 min 1 min 2 min

When you hit week 4, you're going to do three exercise sets as in week 3. Except this time, you're going to reduce the exercise periods to just 1 minute each, followed by 2-minute recovery periods.

Apply the same principles. Take your warm up at a low to moderate intensity. Then turn up the intensity, when you start your first exercise period.

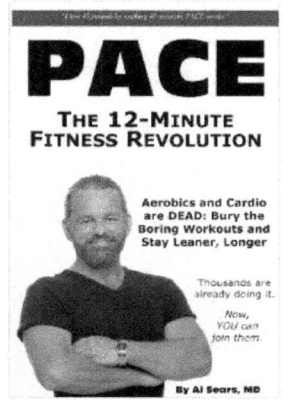

Remember, don't stress yourself. As you decrease the exercise duration, you turn up the intensity. And, by decreasing the duration, it will actually feel easier, as the 4th week progresses.

Here's where to get the **full Pace Program**. It is an excellent way to exercise, for a short time and still get the benefits of greater health and stronger heart.

But, remember to measure your heart beat before and after each exercise period.

Chapter Summary

Exercise is a must for this acne program. It makes you sweat, so you can release more toxins. And even more important is that you will improve your cardiovascular system, and this will make you healthier.

This program starts with a chart that defines what your heart rate should be at the end of your exercise. By increasing the intensity of your exercise daily, you will reach higher heart rates. Eventual you will reach your maximum exercise heart rate for your age.

This exercise is a short exercise, but requires more intense exercising as each day passes.

Chapter 31: Preparing For Your Acne Program

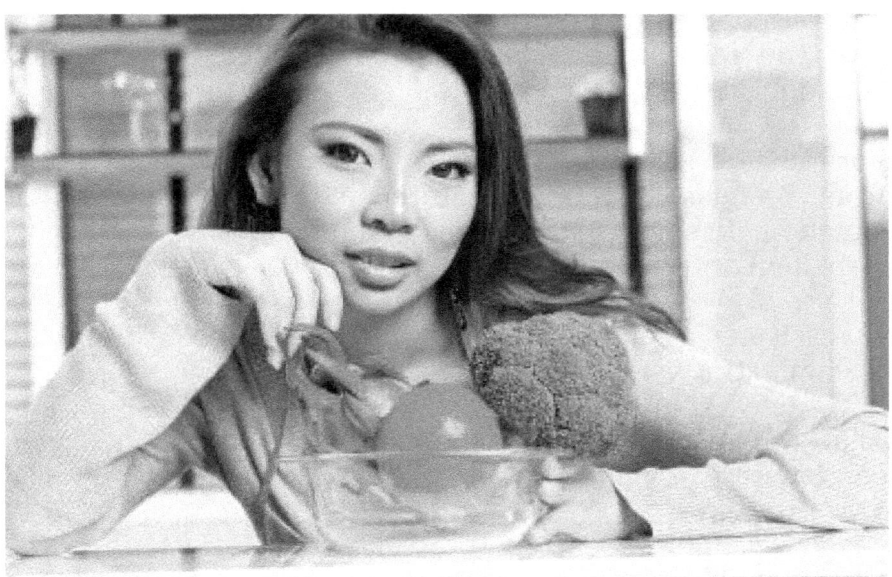

In this chapter, you will find the instructions on how to start preparing for your acne program. You can collect all the products and review certain chapters that you need to get started on this program.

How to Get Started

There many things you can do for acne, and some will work and others will not. What does work for you, may not work for others. This is why there are a lot of products and techniques for acne in this book.

You don't have to use all the information or all the products listed in this book. If you can't afford many of the products, don't worry about it. Use the alternative cheaper products recommended and you will still get results.

If you don't have a specific product, just keep working the program without it. Your body will respond to the various changes that you make and reward you with better looking skin.

The purpose of providing you with a lot of information is to give you ideas and techniques that applied to your life's situation.

For the different steps, there may be many products to choose from. Choose the ones that relate to your condition or situation. In some cases, you may want to skip using a specific step, item or technique.

Do each step as outline and this will give you the best success, in eliminating your acne.

Acne can be a difficult condition to eliminate. But, if you consistently in apply the processes outline here, you will succeed.

Once you have diminished, eliminated, or have your acne under control, you can lessen the supplements that you have to take. But, this should be only because you have a better diet, are eating more fruits and vegetables, and have developed a good lifestyle.

Acne is all about having a body that is out of balance physical and emotionally. To get the physical part back into balance, you need to use nutrition, cleansing, hormonal balancing, elimination channel stabilizing, and facial cleansing.

To get the emotional part back into balance is a difficult process. People for hundreds of years have been searching for approaches to psychological balance.

What is important to realize is you can't keep the same lifestyle that has produced the acne you have.

You need to change the three areas that are important in a good lifestyle – nutrition, emotions, and exercise.

A Plan for Your Acne Program

As you start this acne program, you may be doing 2 or 3 different steps at the same time. This summary will tag those sections that you can do simultaneously.

There are a lot of products that have been recommended. If you are limited on money, chose that route that is less expensive. If you are a good experimenter, you can keep your costs down. Hopefully, you might already have some of these products.

If you can do this program with a partner, you will have more success and will be more motivated. When you get discouraged, your partner may be upbeat and help both of you keep going. But, if you are self-motivated, you will be successful, in this program.

This program will take about 8 to 10 weeks. Each week, you will be given something to do from the previous chapters. When a specific chapter is mention go back and review that chapter and make an outline of what you have to do.

What you have to do each week may seem complicated at first. But, there are some items that will not take you long to do. Just get started and do what you can. You can always repeat a week to solidify your success of this program.

So, let get started.

Products to Buy

The first thing you want to do is buy some of the products you need to get started. So order or buy the following items, if you don't have them. Do this about one to two weeks before you start this program.

Preparation before the First Week of the Program

Products to Order

Order the products you need for this program. These are the first items to buy.

1. Omega-3 Norwegian Fish Oil for men and Primrose oil for women.
2. Digital thermometer
3. Chlorophyll liquid
4. Lemons
5. Glycerin hand soap
6. loose oregano leaf, fresh ginger, green tea, caffeine free
7. melatonin
8. supplements: vitamin A, C, D3, B100, Zinc, Folic acid, Selenium, Chromium, magnesium
9. probiotics
1. digestive enzymes
2. lecithin

Review Chapter 15 for Constipation

Look over Chapter 15: Eliminating Your Constipation. Examine the diet in this chapter and start planning what you will be eating and what food you will be eliminating from your diet. You will be starting this diet, during your first week of this program. So, start buying some of the food to eat during this week. Every day of your first week, make some changes in what you eat. You don't need to make a sudden change in your entire diet.

Do Your Tests First

Once you get the things you ordered, do your testing for your health base line. Test for,

1. transit time
2. candida
3. thyroid

Go back to each chapter to get the details for each test.

Set up a note book to record the reading. You will be doing these tests at different points during this program.

Chapter 32: Acne Program Step by Step

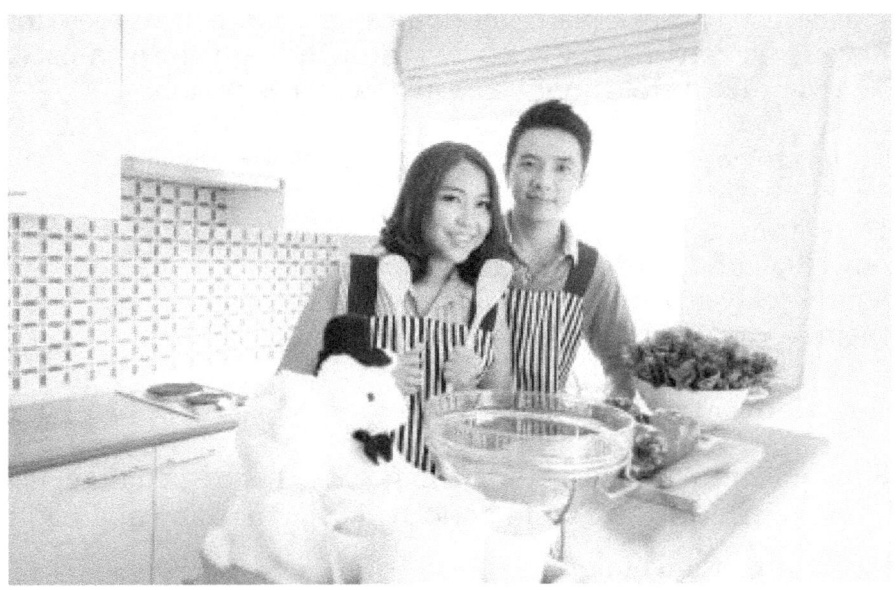

Purpose of this Chapter

In this chapter you will find step by step instructions for doing your acne program. There are 10 weeks for you to follow. Each day in these weeks, will be outlined, so that you know what to do daily.

This is a detailed step by step acne program. You don't have to do every detailed step. This is a guide for you to use the step that you feel comfortable with the products that you have. Make you owe step by step program. Each day do something from the daily list. And you can always go back and do more of the steps when you want to upgrade your program.

These steps will provide you with a direction on how to use all the information, in this book. It gives you a good start, so if you are confused, with all the information provided, you will have a plan to get started.

This plan is a day by day and week by week plan.

It is a fast 10 week plan, but you can go slower. It does not have to be done in 10 weeks. Go through it at your own pace. You may decide to do one week in a two week period.

Things to do Every Day during Your 10 Week Program

Here are the things that you need to do every day or every other day of this program. Incorporate these 8 items below in your weekly acne program. Keep track of when you need to do them.

Supplementation

Supplements are to be taken with meals or before bed time.
- Vitamin D3 3000 to 4500 IU in the morning and night for a total of 6000 to 9000 IU.
- Vitamin B50 or B100
- Vitamin A (water soluble), 25,000 to 30,000 IU
- Vitamin C, buffered 1000mg three times a day
- Vitamin E, 400 IU, two times
- Calcium – magnesium 1000 mg daily
- Zinc 20 to 30 mg
- Selenium 20, to 30 mg
- Fish oil 1500 mg daily
- melatonin

1. Skin Brushing

Brush your skin, with a Loofah during your shower every other day.

2. Mediation Tapes

Listen to your mediation or paraliminal tapes, at least two times a week.

3. Herbal Tea

Drink an herbal tea every day or every other day. Go back to Chapter 19 and look over the list of herbs to use. Here are a few to start with. Use a touch of honey, if you like.

Green tea

Licorice root

Ginger

Cinnamon

Chamomile
Hops

4. Get Fresh Air

Every day go outside for 20 minutes or so to get some air and sunshine.

5. Exercising

Three times a week do your Pace Exercises. You can do them four times a week, if you like. You will be starting out slowly. If you are already exercising, then you can also use the information in exercise Chapter to measure your heart rate.

6. Digestive Enzymes

Start taking digestive enzymes before or after each meal.

7. Melatonin

Take 2 to 4 mg of melatonin every night. You can take more melatonin, if you want up to 12 mg. Just test to see what you need.

First Week of Acne Program

First week, start to make changes in your diet. To change your diet into a healthy one will take a long time, but you need to get started. The information for this diet comes from Chapter **12.** So, go back and review the diet.

A reminder, take a photo of your acne before starting this program.
Day 1 – First you want to look over the chapter on eliminating constipation, and start using the eating habits in that chapter. Continue to eat in this fashion, until you start another step in this program that calls for a different diet.

- Start drinking 6 to 8 glass of water every day.

- Herbal tea counts as water and the water in fruits and vegetables.

Day 2 – look to see what to eat to get more fiber and buy that food.

Day 3 – if you eat a lot of meat back off a slight bit. Every time you eat meat, keep backing off on the amount your eat.

- Eat more salad. Use many different dark-green leaf lettuces and add cucumber, tomato, radish, and many of the other raw vegetables you like. Mix in a salad dressing that contains flax oil, olive oil, and apple cider vinegar.

- If you have been eating a lot of sweets, start backing off little by little. Put in its place a fruit of any kind.

Day 4 – look at your breakfast and start backing off on a heavy breakfast.

- Introduce more fruits during your breakfast.

- Start taking digestive enzymes with before or after each meal.

Day 5 – Drink fruit juices during break times
Day 6 – eat more salads with your meals
Day 7 – introduce eating fish once a week

Remember to do all these things during each week for the next 10 weeks.

1. Start taking 2-4mg melatonin every day from this time forward.

2. Every day of this week start practicing the steps in the skin cleaning Chapter.

3. Exercise 4 times a week using the PACE program in chapter 34.

4. During this week create an herbal mix of chamomile, licorice root, and hops. Drink this tea for three days to five days, during the week.

5. Take vitamin D3 in two doses, morning and night of 3500 to 4000 IU each time for a total of 7,000 to 8,000 IU per day all through this program.

6. Start taking Vitamin C 3000 to 5000 mg per day divided into three doses all through this program.

7. Start taking Vitamin A and B50 or B100

8. Start taking fish oil up to 1500 mg

Second Week Of Acne Program

During this week you will be following Chapter 11: Getting Rid of Parasites and Candida and doing the body cleanse outlined in Chapter 14 or 15, Oxypowder Body Cleanse or Prune Juice Body Cleanse.

You will measure your thyroid temperature chapter 9.
Day 1 – Check that you have all items for your Oxypowder or Prune Juice body cleanse. Be ready to start your cleanse, starting on Wednesday or Day 4 of this week.

- **Order the creams** for the first cleansing method – Salicylic Acid.

- Start drinking herbal teas, for eliminating candida.

- Measure your thyroid temperature, before you get up.

- Then measure your saliva and measure your first urine pH in the morning. Measure urine two hours after lunch.

- Then, measure your saliva, after swishing lemon juice in your mouth. Wait one minute after lemon swishing, to measure your pH.

Day 2 - Measure your thyroid temperature, before you get up.

- Then measure your saliva and first urine pH, in the morning. Measure your urine

  two hours after lunch.

- Measure your saliva, after swishing lemon juice in your mouth.

Day 3 - Measure your thyroid temperature, before you get up.
- Then measure your saliva and first urine pH, in the morning. Measure urine two hours after lunch.

- Measure your saliva, after swishing lemon juice in your mouth. Record all your measurements.

Day 4 – start your body cleansing using Oxypowder or prune juice.

Day 5 – continue your body cleansing
Day 6 – continue your body cleansing
Day 7 - continue your body cleansing. Last day of the cleanse.

Things to do simultaneously, during the second week.

1. Supplementation

2. Skin Brushing

3. Mediation Tapes

4. Herbal Tea

5. Get Fresh Air

6. Exercising

7. Digestive Enzymes

8. Continue using the constipation diet to improve your eating habits. Do this for the first three days of this week before starting your body cleansing. Review your body cleansing the day before the cleanse.

9. Drink the herbal teas and other products for eliminating candida. Do this for the first three days of this week.

Third Week Of Acne Program

In the third week, you will start the first acne cleansing method as outlined in Chapter 22: *Acne Benzoly Facial Cleansing Method.*

and continue targeting parasites, bacteria, and Candida. Follow the instruction as outline in Chapter 11: *Getting Rid of Parasites and Candida.*

Day 1 – Start your first acne cleansing method. When you first get up, drink your chlorophyll drink or lemon drink.

- Do the salicylic acid cleanse, followed by glycolic acid in the morning

- In the evening do the salicylic acid, followed by Benzoyl Peroxide.

- Follow this with lemon juice, aloe vera, and vitamin E

Make sure you are using garlic, onions, and ginger, in all of your meals.

- Make a tea of cinnamon, with a touch of honey or stevia. Drink this every morning for this week.

- Use coconut oil for any cooking that you do.

- Make a tea of green tea, oregano leaf and ginger. Drink one cup per day in the evening.

Day 2 – Take a garlic capsule with every meal, for the next two weeks or add extra garlic in your food.

- Do the salicylic acid cleanse followed by glycolic acid in the morning

- In the evening do the salicylic acid followed by Benzoyl Peroxide.

- Follow this with lemon juice, aloe vera, and vitamin E

Day 3 – Use probiotics every day between meals, for the next month.
- Do the salicylic acid cleanse, followed by glycolic acid in the morning

- In the evening do the salicylic acid, followed by Benzoyl Peroxide.

- Follow this with lemon juice, aloe vera, and vitamin E

*Day 4 - **Continue drinking different teas as listed in Chapter** 11: Eliminating Parasites and Candida.*

- Do the salicylic acid cleanse, followed by glycolic acid in the morning

- In the evening do the salicylic acid, followed by Benzoyl Peroxide.

- Follow this with lemon juice, aloe vera, and vitamin E

Day 5 – Continue changing over to eating more fruits and vegetable juices during the morning. Keep backing off from eating eggs, potatoes, or meat in the morning. Eat this way all during this week. However, try to eat more vegetable juices for breakfast.

- Do the salicylic acid cleanse, followed by glycolic acid in the morning

- In the evening do the salicylic acid, followed by Benzoyl Peroxide.

- Follow this with lemon juice, aloe vera, and vitamin E

Day 6 – During this week start putting apple cider vinegar on your salads.

- Do the salicylic acid cleanse, followed by glycolic acid in the morning

- In the evening do the salicylic acid, followed by Benzoyl Peroxide.

- Follow this with lemon juice, aloe vera, and vitamin E

Day 7 – For stress relief start listening to relaxing music for 30 minutes, or if you bought the paraliminal tapes, start listening to them when you first wake up or during mid-day, if you can.

There is no acne cleansing on this day.

Things to do simultaneously, during the third week

1. Back off on eating sweets, sugar, fructose, milk

2. During this week create an herbal mix of chamomile, licorice root, and lavender. And drink a cup 3-4 times during the week. Rotate with the other herbal teas that are scheduled for you to drink during the week.

3. Place a teaspoon of apple cider vinegar in about 4 oz. of water and drink this 2-3 times a day for the whole week.

4. Supplementation

5. Skin Brushing

6. Mediation Tapes

7. Herbal Tea

8. Get Fresh Air

9. Exercising

10. Digestive Enzymes

Fourth Week of Acne Program

Order your Dr. Schulze's Kidney Teas for next week.

In this week, you will continue doing Chapter 22: Acne Benzoly Facial Cleansing Method.

Also, during this week, you will start practicing your new alkaline diet from

***Chapter** 25: Acne Free With An Alkaline Diet.*

In this diet, you will be using more alkaline foods, so that you can flood your body with alkaline minerals. Now, you can start to repair and balance your body and at the same time get rid of more parasites.

Strive to eat 80% fruits and vegetables and 20% meat, beans, and other acid foods.

Day 1 – measure your saliva and urine pH first thing in the morning, for the next three days as you have in the pasted weeks.

- After your pH tests, drink a chlorophyll and lemon drink. Do this every day this week.

- After your chlorophyll drink wait about 1/2 hour before you have breakfast. Eat a combination of watermelon and other melons.

- Do the salicylic acid cleanse, followed by glycolic acid in the morning.

- In the evening, do the salicylic acid,

followed by Benzoyl Peroxide.

- Follow this with lemon juice, aloe vera, and vitamin E.

Day 2 – After your pH tests, drink a chlorophyll and lemon drink. Only eat fruits, fruit puddings, or fruit shakes, in the morning.

- Do the salicylic acid cleanse, followed by glycolic acid in the morning.

- In the evening, do the salicylic acid, followed by Benzoyl Peroxide.

- Follow this with lemon juice, aloe vera, and vitamin E.

Day 3 – After your pH tests, drink a chlorophyll and lemon drink. For breakfast eat a pudding of papaya, mango, banana, apple and juice of one lemon or grapefruit.

- Do the salicylic acid cleanse, followed by glycolic acid in the morning.

- In the evening, do the salicylic acid, followed by Benzoyl Peroxide.

- Follow this with lemon juice, aloe vera,

  and vitamin E.

Day 4 – for breakfast make a vegetable juice of carrots, celery, spinach, and apples.

- Do the salicylic acid cleanse, followed by glycolic acid in the morning.

- In the evening, do the salicylic acid, followed by Benzoyl Peroxide.

- Follow this with lemon juice, aloe vera, and vitamin E.

Day 5 – Fix a breakfast of guacamole, using avocados, onions, garlic, lemon juice, sea salt and your favorite chili sauce.
- Do the salicylic acid cleanse, followed by glycolic acid in the morning

- In the evening, do the salicylic acid, followed by Benzoyl Peroxide.

- Follow this with lemon juice, aloe vera, and vitamin E.

Day 6 – Drink a herbal tea daily for breaks, such as spearmint, or mint. It's your choice. Most herbs are alkaline.
- Do the salicylic acid cleanse, followed by glycolic acid in the morning

- In the evening, do the salicylic acid followed by Benzoyl Peroxide.

- Follow this with lemon juice, aloe vera, and vitamin E.

Day 7 – Use almonds, walnuts, pine nuts, **pumpkin seeds**, and pecans as break snacks

There is no cleansing on this day.

Things to do simultaneously, during the fourth week
1. Supplementation

2. Skin Brushing

3. Mediation Tapes

4. Herbal Tea

5. Get Fresh Air

6. Exercising

7. Digestive Enzymes

Fifth Week of Acne Program

In this week, you will concentration on kidney cleansing, using the ideas from

Chapter *16: How To Cleanse Your Kidneys.*

and you will do Chapter *23: Second Acne Facial Cleansing Method.*

Order your Dr. Schulze's Liver Teas for next week.

Day 1 – Start the second natural acne cleansing method. This takes about an hour to do, so time this cleanse just before you go to bed. Follow the instruction step by step that are in chapter 26. You can do this morning and night, if you have the time. Otherwise, just do it in the evening.

- Start the Dr. Schulze's kidney cleanse kit. If you do not have this kit, you can drink the kidney cleansing teas in the morning and evening from chapter 19. They can be different teas. But, drink the kidney tonic every morning this week.

Day 2 – Second natural acne cleansing

- Continue with Dr. Schulze's kidney cleanse for 5 days. Or, use the recommended kidney teas and tonics for the next 5 days. Check Chapter **16: How To Cleanse Your Kidneys for the teas you may want to use.**

Day 3 – Second natural acne cleansing
- Dr. Schulze's Kidney cleanse

Day 4 – Second natural acne cleansing
- Dr. Schulze's Kidney cleanse

Day 5 – Second natural acne cleansing
- Dr. Schulze's Kidney cleanse

Day 6 – Second natural acne cleansing
- Dr. Schulze's Kidney cleanse

Day 7 – No acne cleansing today

Things to do simultaneously, during the fifth week

1. Supplementation
2. Skin Brushing
3. Mediation Tapes
4. Herbal Tea
5. Get Fresh Air
6. Exercising
7. Digestive Enzymes

Sixth Week of Acne Program

During this week, your will be doing a liver cleanse, using the information in Chapter 17: Liver Cleansing And Diet. If you don't want to do Dr. Schulze's cleanse, then choose the alternate teas and tonics listed in chapter 20. Continue doing your Second Acne Facial Cleansing.

Day 1 – Second natural acne cleansing
- Start Dr Schulze's liver cleanse

Day 2 – Second natural acne cleansing
- Dr. Schulze's liver cleanse

Day 3 – Second natural acne cleansing
- Dr. Schulze's liver cleanse

Day 4 – Second natural acne cleansing
- Dr. Schulze's liver cleanse

Day 5 – Second natural acne cleansing
- Dr. Schulze's liver cleanse

Day 6 – Second natural acne cleansing
Day 7 – No acne cleansing today
Things to do simultaneously, during the sixth week

1. Supplementation

2. Skin Brushing

3. Mediation Tapes

4. Herbal Tea

5. Get Fresh Air

6. Exercising

7. Digestive Enzymes

8. Continue with your acid alkaline diet by eating those fruits and vegetables that are highest in alkaline minerals.

Seventh Week of Acne Program

During this week, you will be following the body cycles 1, 2 and 3 as outline in Chapter 26: Breakfast Cycle 1 Keeps You Acne Free.

You will also start a new cleansing technique as outlined in Chapter 24: Third Acne Facial Cleansing Method. But, you will alternate with the Second Acne Facial Cleansing method.

During this week you will be reviewing how to get better sleep and doing stress relief using Chapter 18: Stress Relief & Sleep Gives Acne Relief.

Day 1 – Do the Third Acne Facial Cleansing, in the evening. Check your transit time again as outline in Chapter 8: Food Digestion Constipation Transit Time.

1. Use either a chlorophyll or red beet drink. You can take this drink immediately after lunch or dinner. See if you have improved in your transit time.

2. Measure your thyroid temperature, before you get up.

3. Measure your salvia pH first thing in the morning, then check again after a lemon swish.

4. Measure your urine pH, in the morning and afternoon.

Check for candida, using the saliva test with reverse osmosis water and the sesame seed test as outlined Chapter 10: Testing For Candida.
5. Record your results.

Day 2 – Do the **Second Acne Facial Cleansing.**
1. Measure your thyroid temperature, before you get up.

2. Measure your salvia pH first thing in the morning, then check again after a lemon swish.

3. Measure your urine pH, in the morning and afternoon.

During this week, create a herbal mix of chamomile, licorice root, and hops. Use some of the other herbs also that are listed the Chapter 18: Stress Relief & Sleep Gives Acne Relief

4. Use 3-4 herbs to make your own formula.

Day 3 – Do the **Third** Acne Facial Cleansing, in the evening.
1. Use either a chlorophyll or red beet drink. You can take this drink immediately after lunch or dinner. See if your transit time is the same as Day 1.

2. Measure your thyroid temperature, before you get up.

3. Measure your salvia pH first thing in the morning, then check again after a lemon swish.

4. Measure your urine pH, in the morning and afternoon..

Day 4 – Second Acne Facial Cleansing
Day 5 – Third Acne Facial Cleansing, in the evening
Day 6 – Second Acne Facial Cleansing
Day 7 – No acne facial cleanse today

Things to do simultaneously, during the seventh week

1. Supplementation

2. Skin Brushing

3. Mediation Tapes

4. Herbal Tea

5. Get Fresh Air

6. Exercising

7. Digestive Enzymes

Eighth Week of Acne Program

During this week you will be concentrating on Chapter 27: Body Cycle 2 & 3 Keeps You Acne Free. You will be doing body cycle 2 and 3, but you will still be doing body cycle 1. These eating cycles go together.

In addition your will be exploring different herb teas that will help you with your acne and for rebalancing your body. You will be using the information at Chapter 19: Herbal Remedies For Acne.

Again, start doing Chapter 23: Second Acne Facial Cleansing Method. At some point in time, the level of toxins in your body can be handled mostly through the other channels of elimination and not through your skin.

Day 1 – Start your Second Acne Facial Cleansing.
- Read your urine pH and record it.

- Drink a lemon drink or lemon with chlorophyll

- Eat your cycle 1 breakfast. Use high acid binding fruit like watermelon and melons

- Eat your cycle 2 lunch and dinner. Lunch one protein with salad, dinner one carbohydrate with salad

- Drink an herbal tea of your choice before lunch

Day 2 – Do your Second Acne Facial Cleansing.
- Lemon drink with distilled water

- Eat a bowl of unprocessed oat (not 1 minute type), with raisins, banana, and a touch of honey. Use apple juice instead of milk.

- Read your urine pH and record it.

- Eat some fish and salad for lunch

Day 3 – Do your Second Acne Facial Cleansing.
- Read your urine pH and record it.

- lemon drink with distilled water

- Eat cantaloupes or watermelon

Day 4 – Do your Second Acne Facial Cleansing.

Drink a juice of orange, grapefruit and lemon.

Make a fruit smoothie from Chapter 33: Smoothie Recipes For Breakfast.

- Drink an herbal tea of your choice before lunch

Day 5 – Do your Second Acne Facial Cleansing.
- Drink a juice of orange, grapefruit and lemon

- Eat a breakfast of mixed fruits, like mango, kiwis, pineapples, bananas or grapes

- Drink an herbal tea of your choice before

  lunch

- For lunch, eat an avocado sandwich on wheat or rye bread, with romaine lettuce, cucumbers and tomatoes.

- For dinner, eat a protein of your choice, with a big salad.

Day 6 – Do your Second Acne Facial Cleansing.
- Make a pudding from different fruits. Add the fruits into a blender and put just enough apple juice or other juice to get the blender spinning and blending.

- Drink an herbal tea of your choice before lunch.

- Lunch can be some chicken with salad.

- Dinner can be pinto bean vegetable soup.

Day 7 – No facial cleansing today.
Drink a juice of orange, grapefruit and lemon.

- Have a breakfast of grapes, berries, raspberries, strawberries, and apples.

  Use the fruits in season.

- Drink an herbal tea of your choice before lunch.

Things to do simultaneously, during the eighth week
1. Supplementation

2. Skin Brushing

3. Mediation Tapes

4. Herbal Tea

5. Get Fresh Air

6. Exercising

7. Digestive Enzymes

Ninth Week of Acne Program

This week you will continue with the Second Acne Facial Cleansing Method.

During this week you will be concentrating on your stress relief and sleep from Chapter 18: *Stress Relief & Sleep Gives Acne Relief.*

Day 1 – Do the Second Acne Facial Cleansing.
- Listen to a Paraliminal or holosync tape in the morning, when you first wake up. If you have time, you can listen, during the day. These tapes will put you to sleep, if you are tired.

Day 2 – Do the Second Acne Facial Cleansing.
- Listen to a Paraliminal or holosync tape in the morning, when you first wake up. If you have time, you can listen, during the day.

- **Day 3** – Do the Second Acne Facial Cleansing.

- Listen to a Paraliminal or holosync tape in the morning, when you first wake up. If you have time, you can listen, during the day.

Day 4 – Do the Second Acne Facial Cleansing.
- Listen to a para liminal or holosync tape in the morning, when you first wake up.

Day 5 – Do the Second Acne Facial Cleansing.
- Listen to a para liminal or holosync tape in the morning, when you first wake up.

Day 6 – Do the Second Acne Facial Cleansing.
- Listen to a para liminal or holosync tape in the morning, when you first wake up.

Day 7 – This is a rest day.

Things to do simultaneousllly, during the ninth week
1. Supplementation
2. Skin Brushing
3. Mediation Tapes
4. Herbal Tea
5. Get Fresh Air
6. Exercising
7. Digestive Enzymes

Tenth Week of Acne Program

This week you will continue with the **Second Acne Facial Method.**

During this week your will review Chapter 19: Herbal Remedies For Acne. From this chapter, review the different herbal remedies that you can use and choose 3 – 4 different herbals, to use every day. Rotate from one to the

other, to get a variety of nutrients and benefits.

Also, review Chapter 21: *Where To Get Essential Fatty Acids.*

Start using the foods that are high in essential fatty acids. You need to get these fatty acids from food and supplements.

Look over Chapter 20: *Supplements Needed To Eliminate Acne,* **and see what supplement you can now add to your diet that you have not been using.**

Day 1 – Do the Second Acne Facial Cleansing.

Mix a tea containing burdock root, dandelion, yarrow root and Oregon grape root. Drink one cup of this tea 5 days of this week. You may want to change one or more of the herbs, in this drink. For example, use goldenseal or watercress.

- Take your fish oil supplement. For women take borage oil or primrose oil for GLA, every day from now on.

- Add flax seed oil, olive oil, and apple cider vinegar to your salads

- Start adding these foods to your diet, avocados, sesame seeds, pumpkin seeds, walnuts, dark leafy green vegetables (spinach, mustard greens, kale), salmon, albacore tuna

Day 2 – Do the Second Acne Facial Cleansing.
- Drink an herbal tea.

- Start adding these foods to your diet, flaxseed oil, pistachio nuts, olives, olive oil, sunflower seeds, chicken, evening primrose oil, pumpkin seeds, pine nuts

Day 3 – Do the Second Acne Facial Cleansing.

- drink an herbal tea

- Foot spa or tub with herbs

- Use coconut oil for your cooking

Day 4 – Do the Second Acne Facial Cleansing.
- Drink an herbal tea

- Foot spa or tub with herbs

Day 5 – Do the Second Acne Facial Cleansing.
- Drink an herbal tea

Day 6 – Do the Second Acne Facial Cleansing.
- Foot spa or tub with herbs

Day 7 – Do the Second Acne Facial Cleansing.
- Foot spa or tub with herbs

Things to do simultaneously, during the tenth week
1. Supplementation

2. Skin Brushing

3. Mediation Tapes

4. Herbal Tea

5. Get Fresh Air

6. Exercising

7. Digestive Enzymes

If you have a food spa, use it and put herbs into the water. Check out Chapter 20: Supplements Needed To Eliminate Acne, for the instructions. Use the spa four times during the week. Without a foot spa, use a foot tub and add hot water and the herb mixture.

Eleventh Week of Acne Program

This program is now complete. If you still have acne issues and wish to continue this program, you can do it. By this time, you have been exposed to a variety of natural health practices that you can continue. Here what are the most important changes that you should continue using.

1. Continue using the Second Facial Cleansing Method. You don't need to do this every day, but you should do it at least two to three times a week or more, depending on your need.

2. Vary your facial cleansing methods using the other two facials. This way your skin can be stimulated in different ways.

3. Continue eating, using the body cycles. This is where you eat fruits or vegetables or their juices for breakfast. You will be helping to detoxify your body every day.

4. Eat those fruits and vegetables that are high on the acid binding charts. Also eat a variety of produce.

5. Keep taking certain vitamins. You can supplement with a variety of them. But, also take Fish Oil and vary that with flax oil, primrose oil or borage oil. Also, keep up your high vitamin D3 dose, 5000 to 7000. Always take vitamin C, E, A, zinc and selenium. These are the antioxidants, which are needed for acne and they help to control the sebum output. Always eat a salad with your meals. This is where you will get the minerals to neutralize your body's acids. Vegetables give you the fiber you need for colon health.

6. Eat fruits and juices for breakfast for fiber and minerals.

7. Keep drinking green tea, ginger tea, or other herb drinks that you have come to like. Herbs are high in anti-oxidants and special nutrients that give your whole body a nutritional lift.

8. Keep up with your weekly exercise. This is one area that is critical, for your health.

9. Take time to go back through each chapter and see what other health practices you can add to your regime. You will find many recommendations that you did not see the first time around.

Chapter Summary

Here is a 10 weeks step by step program for Your Acne Program. Take each week and follow the individual day steps. You don't have to follow this program exactly as outlined. Make changes according to your needs and your time, products, and food you have available.

What is important is that you do most of what is outlined for each week. Each week builds and prepares you, for the next week.

Thank you for reading and applying this information. This information is for your education, and you assume any risk in applying this information. Study it closely and you decide how you want to use it, to cure your acne.

Final Thoughts

After you finish the ten weeks, and if you need more time to eliminate your acne, go back to day one and start again. But, when you start again, you will be using the diet outlined in

Chapter 26: Breakfast Cycle 1 Keeps You Acne Free

Chapter 27: Body Cycle 2 & 3 Keeps You Acne Free

This is the type of diet you want to be using from now on. Just use the principles outlined in Chapter *25: Acne Free With An Alkaline Diet, with your body cycle diet.*

This diet will help you, with an acid body. You need to keep working on an acid body, since making your body alkaline can take a long time.

Use those foods, supplements, herbs and other nutrients that you have found useful and continue to use them.

Do **only** the second facial, for two or more times per week, if you need to. The third facial you can do once a week.

You now can decide what part of the program you need to do again. You have the information and now you have the power to make major changes in your life. Keep doing all the nutritional principles, you have learned in this program. Eventually, you will have a clear face, free of acne and with super health.

Chapter 33: Breakfast Smoothie Recipes

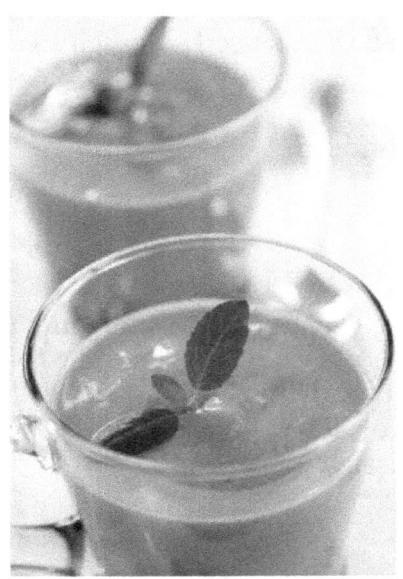

Here is how to build a natural smoothie that can stop constipation, relieve acne, improve your skin and give you more energy. The smoothie base is liquid slurry that can be used to add more natural ingredients. The liquid base can be made from various fresh juices or rice, oat, or almond milks. I stay away from milk since milk creates mucus along the gastrointestinal lining. Choose and mix any of the following liquids and pour them into a blender.

Juices - apple, pineapple, orange, tangerine

Milks - rice dream, oat milk, almond milk

I use a combination of 40% rice dream, 40% almond milk, and 20% apple juice. You can use the combinations you like. Sometimes I might just use all rice dream. Other times I will mix 75% almond milk with 25% fresh apple juice.

All of these juices provide liquid to your colon to help your stop constipation.

Sesame Milk

You can also make sesame milk and use this in your smoothies.

In his book, Blending Magic, Bernard Jensen, Nutritionist, has a really nice recipe for sesame milk.

"I believe that sesame seed is one of our best. It is a wonderful drink for gaining weight and for lubricating the intestinal tract. Its nutritional value is beyond compare, as it is high in protein and minerals. This is the seed that is used so much as a basic food in Arabia and East India.

Blend for 1- 1 1/2 minutes to make smooth,
2 cups of distilled water
1/4 cup of Sesame Seed
2 Tablespoons Soy Milk Powder

In place of 2 cups of distilled water use 1 cup of water and 1 cup of low fat rice dream and leave out the 2 tablespoons of soy milk powder. This will make this drink less fattening. I prefer not to give children soymilk or soy products because of their estrogen mimicking characteristics.

Banana Base

Next I always put in a banana. This gives the liquid a bit more thickness. Also, bananas are high in potassium and other minerals. They contain little fiber and yet do not create constipation when used with other fiber fruits. Use bananas that are not spotted since at this point they are quite ripe and are more fattening.

I freeze bananas so when I am out of fresh ones, I can use frozen ones.

Main Ingredients

Next I choose a fruit that will be the main ingredient. I use strawberries when they are in season, if you have fresh organic fruit, then this is the best way to create your smoothie. What I do is freeze fruit during its season so I can have some of this fruit a bit long than its seasonal run. If the fruit is organic, use the whole fruit without peeling. Whole fruits contain a lot of fiber that will help you stop constipation.

Choose from fruits that are in season.

Avocado
Cantaloupe
Peach, mango, papaya
Pineapple, apricots, apples
Strawberries, blueberries, raspberries
Figs
Dried prunes, peaches, apricots, figs
Nutrients to Add to Your Smoothie Base

Once you have your basic smoothie, you can add other nutrients that will provide you with additional fiber, oil, vitamins, minerals and many other nutrients.

Here is a shortlist of some of the ingredients you can add to your smoothies. Add only 2-3 other ingredients so your smoothie taste doesn't get to complex or unusual. But, can experiment with the different nutrients you wish to add.

Almonds
Beet Juice powder
Black strap molasses
Capra mineral whey
Chia Seeds
Distilled water Ice cubes
Edible dairy whey
Fig Juice syrup
Flaxseed and flax seed oil
Honey, rice syrup
Lecithin granules
Powder vitamin C
Raisins
Rice or oat bran

Sesame seeds
Sunflower seeds, pumpkin seeds
Wheat germ
Making Smoothies

Making smoothies is fun and nutritional. Once you create the base slurry, then you can add many other natural ingredients the will give energy, stop constipation, clear acne, and provide many other health benefits.

Drink a morning smoothie, if you have constipation, or if you have skin problems like acne. Drinking a high fiber smoothie relieves and prevents constipation. It will also provide the nutrients that are necessary for having or keeping a nice clean and smooth skin.

So, here are the six smoothie recipes you can blend.

Apple Smoothie
Apple-Barley Smoothie
Apricot Smoothie
Peach-Rice Dream Smoothie
Pineapple Smoothie
Strawberry Smoothie
Apple Smoothie
Mix in the blender the following.

1-2 small apples cut into wedges
1 banana
1 cup 50:50 rice dream: almond milk
¼ cup or less of raisins soaked overnight
1-teaspoon honey
1-2 cubes of ice
1-teaspoon lecithin granules
2 tablespoons flax seed oil

Start by mixing the banana and the liquids. Then add slices of apples to get the consistency you like. In all of your smoothies add flax seed oil for nice smooth skin. I also add a tablespoon of flax seed straight into the blender, and the blender will chop them   up.

Apple-Barley Smoothie

Mix in the blender the following.

1 cup of sliced apples with peel
1/2 cup of cooked barley
1/4 cup of soaked raisins
1/4 teaspoon of vanilla flavoring
1–1 ½ cup of 50:50 rice dream: almond milk
1-teaspoon lecithin granules
2 tablespoons flax seed oil
Make sure you use the lecithin granules in these smoothies since lecithin helps to break down the flax oil into tiny droplets and makes it more digestible.

Apricot Smoothie

One cup of fresh apricots or dried apricots that were soaked overnight.

juice of 1/2 a lemon
Two oz. of prune juice
one teaspoon or more of oat bran
one teaspoon of mineral whey
one tablespoon of flax seed oil
one tablespoon of lecithin granules

Add a slight amount of distilled water or ice cubes to make the consistency to your liking. This smoothie is good for constipation and acne.

Peach-Rice Dream Smoothie

Mix in the blender:

2 fresh peaches with peel
1-cup rice dream
1/2 banana
1-teaspoon sesame seeds
1-teaspoon sunflower seed
1-tablespoon lecithin granules
2 tablespoons flax seed oil

In place of rice dream you can use almond milk. I now only use almond milk to make my smoothies. Place all of the seeds straight into the blender. This smoothie has plenty of fiber. You may want to increase the amount of sesame and sunflower seeds.

Pineapple Smoothie

Mix the following in a blender.

1-2 cups of fresh pineapples
1/2 cups apple slices
1/4-cup fresh apple juice
1/2-cup almond milk (more or less as needed)
1 banana
1-tablespoon lecithin
2-tablespoons flax seeds
2 teaspoons bran (wheat, oat or rice)

You can add more lecithin if you like. Lecithin does not have a taste. This smoothie is jam packed with fiber.

Strawberry Smoothie

Mix in a blender the following ingredients.

1 banana
1-tablespoon of lecithin granules
1-teaspoon of any type of bran
1 cup or more 50:50 rice dream: almond milk
Now, add strawberries one by one with the blender on until you get the consistency you like.
1-tablespoon flax seeds
1 or 2 tablespoons sunflower seeds
1-teaspoon sesame seeds
1 tablespoon of flax seed oil

You can add liquid minerals or vitamins to these smoothies and give them an additional nutritional value.

There you have the smoothies that I make. Start making and drinking them and see the health benefits that you'll get.

Chapter 34: More Breakfast Recipes

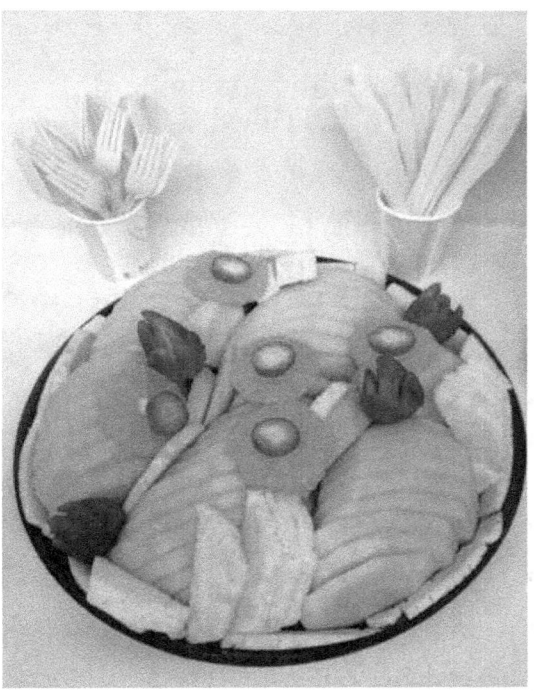

Breakfast Recipes

Here is a list of breakfast recipes for cycle 1 that you can use, in the morning or any time you need a snack. Adjust the ingredients, for the number of people eating.

If you don't have some of the fruits in these recipes, use the ones you have.

Breakfast Pudding

> 5 large dates, pitted

> 1 apple, quartered and cored

1 large frozen banana

Several sections of orange, to taste

Place all ingredients into a blender. Add a bit of apple juice, to get the blender started.

Peaches and Blueberries with a Melon Bowl
4 peaches, peeled and cubed

1 cup blueberries

2 small cantaloupes, halved and seeded

With a spoon or knife, cut up the cantaloupe into small pieces and place them in a bowl, with the other fruits.

Pumpkin Applesauce Pudding

1 cup applesauce

¾ cup pumpkin puree

¼ cup raisins

Ground cinnamon, to taste

Ground nutmeg, to taste

Ground allspice, to taste

Combine all the ingredients in a bowl.

Fruit Salad
Bananas

Kiwis

Mandarin oranges

Pineapple

Apples

Fresh lemon or lime juice

Cut up the fruits and place them in a bowl. You can use other fruits that are in season.

Smoothies

Apple Berry Smoothie

> 1 cup apple juice
>
> 2 apples, peeled, quartered, and cored
>
> ½ cup fresh or frozen blueberries
>
> ½ cup blackberries
>
> 1 medium fresh or frozen banana
>
> 2 dates, pitted

Blend all ingredients, in a blender for one minute.

Banana Peach Drink

> 1 cup apple juice or orange juice
>
> 1 large fresh or frozen banana
>
> 2 ripe peaches, peeled, pitted, and cubed
>
> Fresh strawberries

Blend all ingredients, in a blender for one minute.

Coconut Smoothie

> 1 cup regular or light coconut milk
>
> 1 tablespoon maca powder
>
> 1 tablespoon coconut oil
>
> 1 tablespoon ground flax seeds
>
> 1 teaspoon alcohol-free vanilla extract
>
> ¼ teaspoon almond extract
>
> ¼ teaspoon stevia powder
>
> 8-10 ice cubes

Blend all ingredients, in a blender for one minute.

Fruit Shake

8 ounces orange or apple juice

1 medium banana

½ cup frozen diced peaches (purchased or frozen fresh)

Use any other fruit or combination of fruits that you like.

Strawberry Banana Smoothie

3 cups fresh strawberries

2 medium frozen bananas

1 cup fresh young coconut water

2 tablespoons raw hulled hemp seeds or ground flax seeds.

Blend all ingredients, in a blender for one minute.

Snacks between Meals

Avocado Dressing

4-6 ripe medium avocados

¼ cup fresh lime juice

¼ cup fresh lemon juice

½ teaspoon powdered garlic

1/3 cup olive oil

Water, as needed for consistency

Salt and pepper, to taste

Mix all ingredients in a bowl until avocados is smooth and not extra chunky.

Banana Avocado Snack

2 medium bananas, sliced

2 medium avocados, sliced

Squeeze of fresh lemon or lime juice

Salt to taste

Mix all ingredients in a bowl, until bananas and avocados are smooth and not extra chunky.

Guacamole

8-10 ripe medium avocados

2 tablespoons ground cumin

1 tablespoon garlic, minced

1 tablespoon ground coriander

¼ cup fresh lime juice

1/8 cup fresh lemon juice

2 large tomatoes, finely chopped

Mix all ingredients in a bowl, until avocados is smooth and not extra chunky. Cut this recipe down if you have less people to feed.

Tomato Basil Soup for Breakfast or Snack

5 large tomatoes (about 2 pounds), quartered

1 bunch fresh basil, chopped

2 cups vegetable broth

2 cloves garlic

2 teaspoon olive oil

2 tablespoons balsamic vinegar

Salt and pepper, to taste

Avocado chunks or sautéed eggplant, for garnish

You can eat this hot or cold. If you want to eat it hot, place all these ingredients into a pot and heat for 10 minutes.

Salads

California Morning Salad
1 somewhat firm avocado, diced

1 cucumber, diced

1 jalapeño chile pepper, sliced into thin rings

1 (3.8-ounce) can sliced olives

Juice from 1 lemon

Juice from 1 lime

¼ cup olive oil

Mix all ingredients into a bowl and toss.

Grapefruit with Avocado Salad
1 grapefruit, cut into segments and ¼ cup juice reserved

1 avocado, sliced or diced

¼ cup olive oil

¼- ½ teaspoon kosher salt

1 teaspoon Dijon mustard

Black pepper and black salt, to taste

Mix in a bowl and eat for breakfast or as a snack.

Banana Breakfast Pudding
1 medium ripe banana

6 dates, soaked in water for up to 30 minutes

2 to 3 peaches, pitted, or meat and water from 1 young coconut

2 teaspoon alcohol-free vanilla extract

1 teaspoon ground cinnamon

Agave nectar, to taste

Blend all Ingredients

Chapter 35: Product Resources

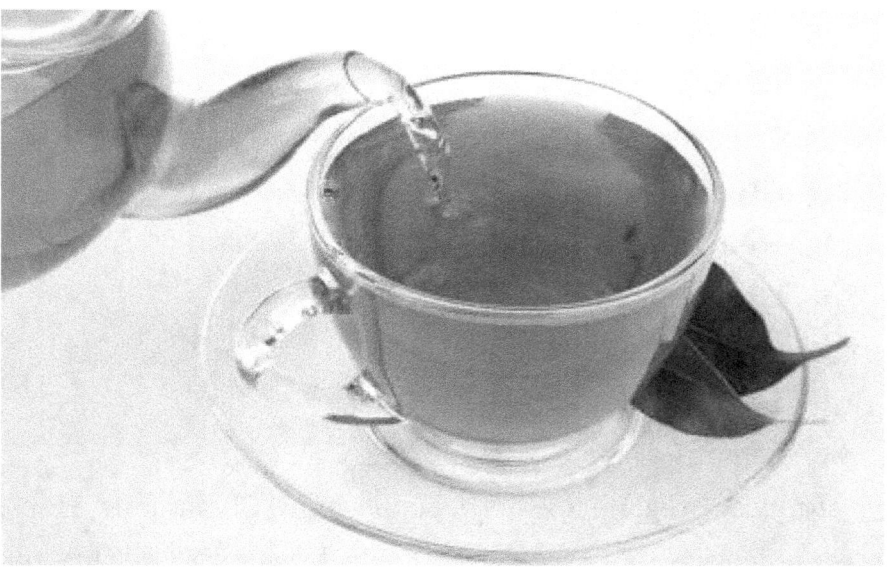

Here is a list of products mentioned in this book. There are many that you will need, to complete this program. However, there are some that you will not need. As you review this program, you can decide, which ones you can buy. Review each chapter to see, which products you have and which ones you want to use.

1. **5 HTP time release**
2. **Glycolic Acid**
3. **Benzoyl Peroxide**.
4. **Calcium Bentonite Clay**
5. **Calcium-magnesium**
6. **Charcoal Activated**
7. **Chlorophyll liquid**

8. **Digestive enzymes**

9. **Digital thermometer**

10. **Dr. Foster's blend**s of jojoba-tree tea oil

11. **Dr. Schulze's Kidney**

12. **Dr. Schulze's Liver**

13. **Garlic capsules**

14. **Glycerin soap**

15. **Hemisync tapes**

16. **Holosync tapes**

17. **Krill Oil, Neptune**

18. **Lecithin**

19. Lemons

20. loose oregano leaf herb, peppermint, Chamomile, Hops, Licorice root, Wormwood, Black walnut, Oregano oil, Peppermint, Rosemary, Olive leaf extract, Grape fruit seed extract, Lavender, Kava Kava, goldenseal, burdock, yarrow, eucalyptus, dandelion root, kelp

Mountain Rose's Herbs

Oregon's Wild Harvest Organic Herbs

21. **Melatonin Sublingual**

22. Olive oil

23. **Omega-3 Norwegian Fish Oil for men**

24. **Oxypowder or Mr. Oxygen OxyFlush**

25. **Pace Exercise Program**

26. **Paraliminal tapes**

27. **Primrose oil for women**

28. **Probiotics**

29. **Rich's MSM Lotion**

30. **Salicylic Acid**

31. **Selenumune Designer Energy - Thyroid**

32. **Scotty's Acne Cream**

33. Supplements: vitamin A, C, **vitamin D3,** B100, Zinc, Folic acid, Selenium, Chromium,

34. **systemic enzymes, Vitalzym**

35. Tea bags of green tea caffeine free

36. **Tree tea oil**

37. Tree tea oil with jojoba oil

38. **Vitex**

Chapter 36: The Author

Christopher Teller is a nutritional consultant educated in the United State in Nutrition. He received his nutritional Certificate from Bauman College: Holistic Nutrition and Culinary Arts, in Berkeley, California.

RESOURCE PAGE

Here are some of the other kindle e-books about natural remedies that he recommends. Here is a list of kindle or paperback books that you might find interesting.

Natural Remedy Books

If you need support or want to promote any of his e-books, please contact him at rss41@yahoo.com. He looks forward to hearing from you.

Here's to creating better health and happiness.